PREGNANCY ANI

MARGARET ROBERTS HERB SERIES

A herbal approach to
Pregnancy and
Baby Care

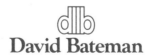

David Bateman

Originally published by Jonathan Ball Publishers.
This edition published in 1990 by David Bateman Ltd,
'Golden Heights', 32–34 View Road, Glenfield,
Auckland 10, New Zealand

Reprinted 1992

ISBN 1 86953 022 5

A David Bateman book
Printed in Hong Kong by Colorcraft

Contents

Foreword

Probably the most important time in your child's life is in the womb. Your health, and thus the health of your unborn baby, will form the foundation for his or her future – and what greater gift can we give our children than that of perfect health? When I was pregnant with my first child, my grandmother gave me this advice: 'Do all you can to be in perfect health. Eat wisely, drink wisely, rest wisely and think wisely, and create within you the picture of a perfect child – no matter be it boy or girl – a perfect, bonny, healthy child is all that counts.'

This, therefore, is what this little book is about. I hope to give you some ideas, borne of my own experiences in carrying and bearing three children, to help you have a healthy baby and to keep him that way in his first years in the world through using natural foods and herbs.

Before you begin, however, I must offer a word of caution. Always work with your doctor and never diagnose anything yourself. Ask your doctor's advice, keep him or her notified of what you are eating, how you are feeling and, once the baby is born, anything that worries you about yourself or him.

The recipes I give, the guidelines to healthy eating and the treatments for common everyday ailments in both mother and child are the results of long years of working with herbs and health-giving food. I offer no better advertisement than my own three children, Peter, Gail and Sandra, who are all healthy, vibrant individuals. I have them to thank for all the things they taught me and it is because of them that I am able to write this book. They suffered my experiments, my inexperience and my struggles to make them into healthy beings. Peter's allergies and illnesses as a baby sparked off my interest in herbs and intensified my search for natural alternatives. His problems turned my thinking away from antibiotics and chemicals to natural medicines. He changed my outlook and set my feet on the path lined with herbs. I used herbs to soothe his cough, clear his nappy rash, calm his sleep and flavour his food. It was a frantic time, with fear and worry as my close companions. In and out of hospital, I took him to every doctor I knew and he baffled them all. Allergy tests showed dogs, grasses, horses and house dust as his greatest irritants. We lived on a farm – how ever did you get rid of those? Finally, a wise paediatrician suggested that I look with utmost care to his diet and I read up on herbs and experimented with all I could and eventually emerged with a healthy son, and the comfort of much knowledge. My two daughters reaped the benefits of my studies, and it is with a thankful heart that I share with you my children's attainment to health and well-being.

My thanks go to Debbie King for typing and putting the manuscript in order and to the discerning and meticulous eye of my editor, Alison Lowry. I value her guidance, her commonsense and her eye for detail.

Conversion Tables

Volume

mℓ to Teaspoons	mℓ to Tablespoons	mℓ to Cups	mℓ to Pints
1 mℓ = $\frac{1}{4}$ tsp	12,5 mℓ = 1 tbsp	60 mℓ = $\frac{1}{4}$ cup	570 mℓ = 1 pt
2 mℓ = $\frac{1}{2}$ tsp	25 mℓ = 2 tbsp	80 mℓ = $\frac{1}{3}$ cup	1,1 ℓ = 2 pts
5 mℓ = 1 tsp	37,5 mℓ = 3 tbsp	125 mℓ = $\frac{1}{2}$ cup	1,7 ℓ = 3 pts
10 mℓ = 2 tsp	50 mℓ = 4 tbsp	180 mℓ = $\frac{3}{4}$ cup	2,3 ℓ = 4 pts
15 mℓ = 3 tsp		250 mℓ = 1 cup	
20 mℓ = 4 tsp		500 mℓ = 2 cups	
		750 mℓ = 3 cups	
		1 litre = 4 cups	

Mass

Grams to Ounces	g/kg to Pounds
30 g = 1 oz	450 g = 1 lb
60 g = 2 oz	900 g = 2 lb
125 g = 4 oz	1,4 kg = 3 lb
250 g = 8 oz	1,8 kg = 4 lb
	2,3 kg = 5 lb

Oven Temperatures	Celsius (°C)	Fahrenheit (°F)
Very cool	100-120	210-250
Cool	130-160	270-320
Moderate	170-180	340-360
Moderately hot	190-210	370-410
Hot	220-240	430-460
Very hot	250 +	480 +

Congratulations – you're pregnant!

The ancient Greeks took particular care of their child-bearing women and perhaps we could take a few lessons from their philosophy today. A few months before conception, women were taken to a special place of tranquillity. Here their diets were watched over by trained 'nurses' and they listened to beautiful music, were offered only pure foods and drank fresh spring water and goats' milk. Their husbands could visit them constantly but the women remained in the peaceful environment (no interfering mother-in-laws, family or friends!). Then, once they were pregnant, they spent the next nine months there, bathing in the natural pools in those beautiful surroundings, walking in the gardens that were exquisitely laid out with statues, fountains and fragrant flowers. They continued their diet of natural foods and drinks, while their nurses soothed their backs and stretching bodies with fragrant oils. No harsh sounds or words or anxieties were allowed to disturb them. What an enchanting time to allow one's baby to grow within those unstressed bodies, but how impractical for today's woman! There are few of us who could lay claim to that sort of time, or are able to escape life's daily stresses, or indeed afford such luxury.

So often a pregnancy is not even planned and no time is available to think about diet or a change in lifestyle. Still – better late than never! As soon as you know that you are pregnant, for the sake of your own health and that of the life now within you, the following important steps should be taken.

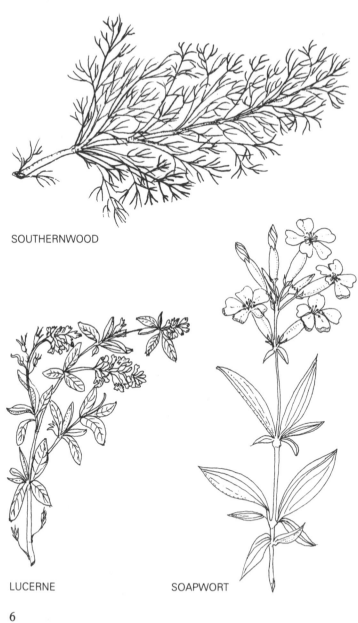

SOUTHERNWOOD

LUCERNE

SOAPWORT

6

AVOID

- all refined, processed, treated, tinned, stabilised, 'junk' foods
- all alcohol
- all tranquillisers, aspirin, pep-pills, sleeping pills etc. (Discuss any medication you may be on with your doctor.)
- fad dieting
- stimulants, eg caffeine-rich beverages, artificial creamers in teas, instant coffee
- curries, chutneys and condiments. The hot spicy flavourings will increase the chances of heartburn and digestive discomfort

INCLUDE IN YOUR DIET

- natural, unrefined foods
- wholewheat meal and bran in homemade bread (learn to bake your own)
- raisins, dates and honey if you have a sweet tooth, rather than sweets and chocolates
- plenty of fresh fruit and vegetables
- increased fluids in the form of mild herb teas, pure, fresh water and milk.
- plain yoghurt and buttermilk
- vitamins. Ask your doctor to advise you on increasing your vitamin supplements; Vitamin C and Vitamin B Complex are essential.
- proteins (meat, fish, poultry, milk, eggs, nuts, butter, cheese and beans – kidney, haricot, butter, sugar, lima, soya etc).

Basic menu for healthy eating in pregnancy

BREAKFAST

Fruit – one portion of any of the following: pawpaw (excellent to keep the stomach working well), mango, orange (with a little of the white rind), grapefruit, peach, apple, grapes, apricots, figs or strawberries.

One helping of homemade *muesli*, with hot or cold milk.

Yoghurt – about 125 ml.

Slice of *wholewheat toast*, with a little honey, Marmite or cream cheese.

Herb tea – lemon balm, mint or peppermint all make a delicious start to the day. Take three or four fresh leaves and pour over 250 ml boiling water. Stand, steep and strain before drinking. Sweeten to taste with a little honey, or add a squeeze of lemon juice.

MID-MORNING

A cup of *buttermilk* or plain unsweetened *yoghurt*.

A glass of whole *milk* or a piece of fresh *fruit*. (Add a little fresh wheatgerm, about 10 ml daily, to your milk.)

LUNCH

A portion of lean *meat*, *chicken* or *fish*

8

A *green salad* – include, for example, lettuce, spinach, beetroot tops or dandelion greens. Top with a health salad dressing: mix 250 ml oil, 250 ml freshly squeezed lemon juice and 250 ml honey in a screw-top jar. Seal and shake well. Add 12,5-25 ml of either chopped thyme, mint, sage, oregano or tarragon.

Steamed *vegetables*, seasoned with lemon juice and a light sprinkling of thyme or marjoram or tarragon.

Baked *potato*, split open and with a little cream or cottage cheese, mixed with chopped chives or parsley, pushed into it.

For dessert, fresh whole or mashed *fruit*, with or without a little yoghurt on top.

A glass of fresh *milk* if no yoghurt is eaten.

MID-AFTERNOON

Freshly squeezed *fruit juice*, fruit shake or *herb tea*.

DINNER

Homemade *vegetable soup*.

Poached or boiled *egg* with wholewheat bread and cottage cheese, OR
Cold *chicken* or *beef*, with steamed vegetables or salad with sprouts.

Fresh *fruit*.

A glass of milk, warmed and sweetened with a little honey, just before bedtime.

VITAMINS

During pregnancy and while you are breastfeeding your baby extra vitamins are essential if you want to maintain peak health for both of you. Consult your doctor here; he will probably recommend a supplement of Vitamin B Complex and Vitamin E. Your vitamin intake needs to be carefully balanced in these important months. Be warned though – too much is as bad as too little, so do take your doctor's advice.

If you are able to plan ahead, Vitamin E can be used for some months before pregnancy. It helps keep the body in shape as it is known to firm up muscle tone. It is also known to firm up sagging breasts and stomach muscles after the baby is born, as well as varicosities. Wheatgerm and wheatgerm oil are good sources of Vitamin E and an easy and healthy way of increasing its intake in your diet. Make sure to buy a reputable brand and see that it is fresh. Keep it in the fridge once you have started using it.

Vitamin C fights infections, keeps skin and muscle tone in tip-top condition, and in fact is essential to one's well-being, especially during the winter months. Vitamin C will actually give you an energy boost – 500 mg at midday will see you into your evening activities if you feel yourself flagging. Do not take Vitamin C after 4 pm however.

These two vitamins are freely available on the market. Between your chemist and your doctor work out a suitable programme for yourself.

CONSTIPATION

Constipation can become a very real problem for the expectant mother, but it is a problem which can so easily be sorted out through correct eating. It is essential that you have at least one bowel movement a day. Toxins and waste need to be cleansed from your system in order to keep blood and body fluids moving and bringing nourishment to your unborn child. Prevent constipation by:

10

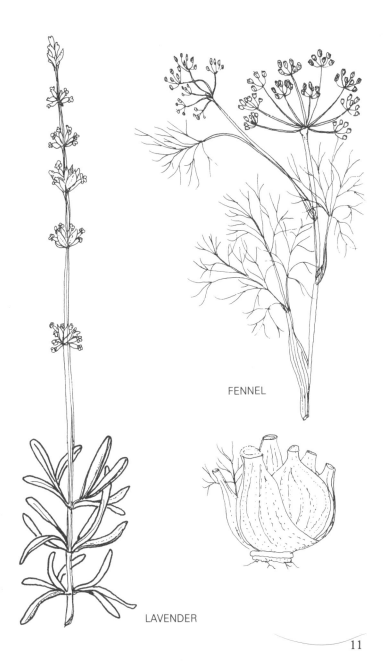

FENNEL

LAVENDER

11

- drinking *water*, at least four glasses a day. It should be fresh and pure, without juice or flavouring of any kind.

- including *roughage* in your diet, eg wholewheat bread, bran, breakfast muesli.

- eating *fruit*. Pawpaw, prunes soaked overnight in water, and grapes all have laxative properties.

- including *oil* in the diet. Sunflower or maize oil are easiest to digest. Use them in stirfry dishes and in salad dressings.

If constipation is already a problem for you, try the following recipe:

25 ml digestive bran
25 ml sunflower oil
25 ml skimmed milk powder

Mix together and add to your breakfast muesli, porridge, mashed fruit or yoghurt. This recipe has proved to be infallible. Take it each morning until your bowel movements are easy and regular again. If you are chronically constipated, consult your doctor immediately. Avoid any harsh laxatives during pregnancy.

EXERCISE

Pregnancy is an important period to keep the body trim, supple and vigorous. Antenatal classes should be a time of pleasure for expectant mothers. Encourage your baby's father to come along too and get fit alongside you. It will give him a chance of getting to know the changes your body is undergoing and to appreciate the aches and pains you may experience. This is a good opportunity for couples to exercise together and to support each other.

Antenatal classes should include back exercises, pelvic floor exercises (to strengthen those muscles used in labour) and, most important, breathing exercises. A good instructor will use rhythm and music and by the end of the class the mothers-to-be will emerge flushed and radiant, circulation moving and stiffness gone.

These are joyful classes and I urge you to attend them. Find out about them from your doctor, hospital or clinic, or join a gym which offers such classes. Take care, though, that you have a qualified person to teach you for this is a crucial time in your life and that of your baby, and wrong exercising can do untold damage. Do the exercises at home too, particularly the breathing ones. These will keep your lungs strong and help you when you go into labour.

RELAXATION

Relaxation is as important as exercise during pregnancy. A midday rest is ideal, but as this blissful activity is often not possible, especially for the mother who has other small children, catnaps or just moments of putting your feet up and doing some deep breathing exercises every now and then will have to suffice. If you *can* manage a midday lie-down, try lying in the following position. (During all three of my pregnancies I found this the most comfortable position of all and, as the baby grows, almost the only really peaceful way of lying.)

Turn on your side, placing your head on a not too high pillow. Turn the upper shoulder towards the pillow, arm bent and hand tucked beneath it. Twist the hips so that the upper bent leg rests on another pillow. The leg underneath should be straight or slightly flexed. The arm underneath should be straight too. The pelvis and abdomen are thus supported on the bed and the weight is lifted.

You will find that the baby enjoys this position too; mine kicked vigorously the minute I wanted to sleep, but I found it so comfortable I didn't mind! Practise in the early months to get used to resting this way so that with the increased weight you will find it easy to relax into. Twenty minutes lying comfortably on your bed, supported by pillows, and breathing deeply will help you unwind.

I found, too, that quiet, restful music would have a calming effect on both myself and the baby. (I also played gentle music while I breastfed in a comfortable armchair and I found my babies had hardly any wind.) Try to avoid all loud, jarring sounds and heavy beats. Believe it or not, peaceful sounds make peaceful babies.

SLEEP

Sleep during pregnancy is vital for both you and the unborn baby. Make the most of it – it is probably the last chance you will have for an undisturbed eight hours for quite some time! In my very first pregnancy I created the 'peace pillow' and I found that I slept well and always woke with a clear head. This is a small pillow filled with calming herbs such as lavender, mint, scented geranium or rose petals. It is light and easy to carry about with you and it also soothes aching backs or stiff necks. Twenty-five years later I still advocate the use of a peace pillow, pregnant or not, for restful sleep. In fact I am never without one. It is easy and pleasurable to make:

PEACE PILLOW

Inner lining: Take a piece of polyester cotton, 30 cm × 20 cm, and sew up into a rectangle, leaving a 12 cm opening along one side. I sew a double row of stitches as this will keep the finer herbs from escaping.

Cover: Make the cover 1 cm bigger all the way round, with a flap of 8 cm. Choose a pretty print in a soft voile or polyester cotton. Use a fabric that does not crease and will wash easily.

14

Make it up as you would a pillow case and edge with lace.

Filling: Half fill your pillow with soft foam chips (usually about 6 cups of foam, depending on how firm you like it). Meanwhile lay your herbs out to dry. Place them on a newspaper in the shade, using enough herbs to make two cups of leaves and flowers. The following filling is a beautifully fragrant one:

2 cups scented geranium leaves
3 cups rose petals
1 cup peppermint leaves
1 cup rosemary leaves
2 cups lavender leaves and flowers
1 cup minced dried lemon peel and pips
2 sticks cinnamon, broken into small pieces
½ cup whole cloves
lavender oil

Mix dry ingredients and add a few drops of oil. Store in a tightly sealed crock or jar. Shake daily. After 10 days add a little more oil until you are satisfied with the fragrance. Store for another week, then turn in the foam chips and mix well.

Stuff the inner case of your pillow with this fragrant mixture. Place it inside your outer pillow case and enjoy the pillow's beautiful comfort and scent. When the aroma starts to fade, turn the contents out into the crock again, add a few drops of lavender oil, shake daily for two days, then return the mixture to your pillow. Add a little fresh lavender or rosemary if you like.

I have kept one of my babies' tiny lawn pillow cases for years. After a particularly hard day, when I've been too tense or rushed, I go into the garden in the cool of the evening and pick a bunch of leaves from my rose scented geranium, some lavender leaves and a few flowers and a few sprigs of rose-

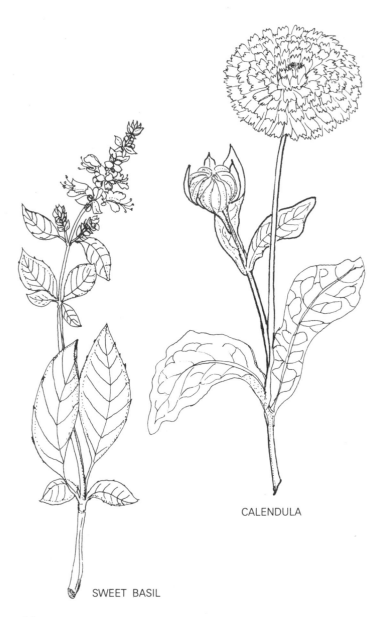

CALENDULA

SWEET BASIL

mary. Sometimes a little lemon verbena goes in too. I strip these leaves from their twigs and push them into the pillow case. I bruise the soft bundle a little and tuck it behind or beside my big pillow. I always sleep soundly and wake much refreshed – what better sleeping pill! The leaves keep for two or three days, after which I shake them out onto newspaper and dry them for adding to pot-pourris.

Another way of unwinding and relaxing after a hard day is to pick a bunch of fresh scented geranium leaves, lavender leaves and flowers, and some mint. Bruise them slightly and place them in a big bowl next to your bed. You will find that you sleep very well that night.

BATHING

Very few things can beat a warm bath for relaxing and un-winding. Living in a very hot part of the country when I was pregnant, I found I sometimes needed to bathe both morning and evening during the summer, or at least freshen up with a brisk, lukewarm shower. At the end of the day, however, a soak in a herb-scented bath is the easiest way of ensuring a good night's rest.

Bath herbs can be varied: lemon balm (melissa), the lavenders, the scented geraniums, the mints, rosemary, sage, rose petals, calendula, violets (leaves and flowers), oatmeal (for itchy skin), thyme, jasmine or honeysuckle will all restore and revive. For further herbal baths, see *Herbs for Health and Beauty* in the Margaret Roberts Herb Series.

SKIN

During pregnancy your skin needs especial care. Some women get away without any of those silvery lines over the abdomen, hips, buttocks and breasts which pregnancy causes. There are, however, some precautions you can take to avoid them. For a start, the increased intake of Vitamin C aids the

17

elasticity of the tissues. During my own pregnancies I took 1000 mg a day and I never had a mark, even though my first two were very big babies.

Comfrey cream with Vitamin E is available at most health shops or chemists. This cream can be rubbed into the skin every evening after your bath to prevent stretchmarks. The following two rubs are also effective.

ALL PURPOSE MASSAGE OIL

1 sprig rosemary
1 sprig chamomile leaves and flowers
medicinal olive oil (available at chemists)
Vitamin E capsules

Infuse rosemary and chamomile in the bottle of oil for three or four days. Strain through muslin or a fine sieve and, to a 500 g bottle, add four Vitamin E capsules (pierce the soft capsule and squeeze out the contents). Put through a blender and massage the resulting oil into the skin, a little at a time. This is also a wonderful massage for cuticles and cracked skin around heels and toes, as well as rough patches on knees and elbows.

Wheatgerm oil used as a massage oil is also excellent. For three days infuse a sprig of rosemary in it for extra healing over taut skin.

HOMEMADE COMFREY CREAM

125 ml aqueous cream
125 ml anhydrous lanolin
250 ml chopped fresh comfrey leaves
125 ml chopped fresh comfrey root

In a double boiler melt all the ingredients together, stirring frequently. Cover and simmer on a low heat for thirty minutes. Discard the leaves and root. Then, while still hot, strain through a fine sieve and ladle into a sterilised jar with a good tight lid. Massage the cream into stomach and breasts during pregnancy, as well as post-natally.

This cream is also excellent for toughening the nipples in preparation for breastfeeding. It will soothe cracked, sore nipples too. Remember, though, to wash nipples thoroughly with warm, soapy water before each feed.

MORNING SICKNESS

Some fortunate women breeze through the early months of pregnancy without even feeling queazy, while others battle constantly with nausea and morning sickness. If at all possible, however, I would strongly advise you never to take medicines and treatments for morning sickness as these first weeks are critical in the life of that tiny foetus inside you and so much can harm it. Try rather to use natural means and treatments and try to remember that at the very most morning sickness will only last three months. There are a few tried and tested methods of bringing relief.

DR BACH'S RESCUE REMEDY

This 'wonder drop' contains a Harley Street specialist's five herbs, all of them anti-shock. A few drops on the tongue at frequent intervals (every few minutes if necessary) will quickly ease the nausea. Rescue Remedy is available at health stores and some pharmacies. It is a lifesaver for so many things – no one should ever be without it.

LEMON JUICE

Never underestimate the humble lemon. A little fresh lemon juice squeezed into a glass of cold water and sipped frequently, will ease the symptoms of morning sickness. If yours is a winter pregnancy, lemon juice in hot water is comforting

19

and as effective. In summer, add a bit of ice or suck an ice cube while sipping the juice.

HERB TEAS

The following herb teas are soothing and refreshing. They will all help to reduce the nauseous feeling of morning sickness. A standard brew is made as follows:

60 ml fresh herb
250 ml boiling water

Pour the water over the herb. Stand, steep for three minutes, then strain. Cool slightly and add honey to sweeten if desired. Never put milk in herb teas. *In pregnancy use slightly less herb than the standard amount. Never use more than 60 ml herb.* If using dried herbs, the standard measurement is 2-5 ml herb to 250 ml boiling water. Stand and steep for four minutes, then proceed as for fresh herbs.

Basil, thyme, ginger and mint are all effective as teas for combating morning sickness in pregnancy.

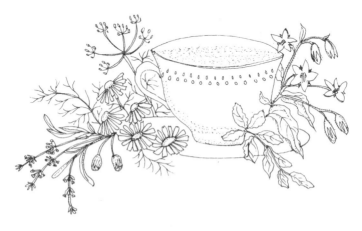

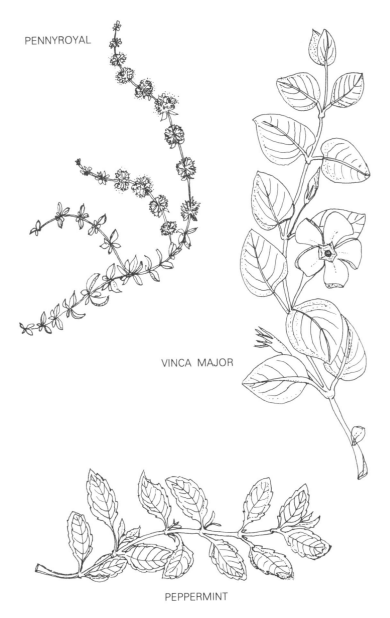

PENNYROYAL

VINCA MAJOR

PEPPERMINT

21

Suitable Herbs for Pregnant Women and the Newborn

Many of the following herbs can be taken in the form of a herb tea. How to make a standard brew is described in the previous chapter and instructions should be followed carefully. Herb teas are health giving and they can also effectively treat a number of ailments. They are beneficial both during and after pregnancy and the herbs listed hereunder will give you some ideas to try out for yourself. First, however, a word of caution: do not overdo things by suddenly drinking vast quantities of herb teas. Tell your doctor what you intend including in your diet and why. Be absolutely sure of the identity of the plant before you use it.

Asparagus (Asparagus officinalis)
Ideally, the wild asparagus is the plant packed with the most minerals and vitamins, but for the city dweller it is almost impossible to find. The next best thing is fresh asparagus tips bought from your greengrocer or, if it is not in season, tinned asparagus will also do. These spears still have some of the vitamins and minerals needed for easing kidney and bladder ailments. The water in which the asparagus is boiled can be used as a tea for clearing kidneys; eat the spears too. If using tinned asparagus, the liquid can be drunk and the spears eaten.

Barley (Hordeum pratense)

Barley makes probably the most useful detoxifying tea known. It is a blood cleanser, a blood cooler, a healer of the internal organs (particularly the kidneys) and a remarkable corrector of kidney ailments. Alternated with asparagus tea, barley water will quickly ease any kidney problems. It is rich in iron, in the B vitamins and in all the minerals, making it excellent for both pregnancy and post-natal diets. Make your own *barley water* as follows:

Boil 500 ml barley in 2 ℓ water. (Use whole barley that is still untreated if you can — it is often available in supermarkets and health shops; otherwise use pearl barley.) Cover and simmer gently for approximately 40 minutes or until the grains are tender. Stand and cool, keeping covered. Then strain off the water and save the rice-like grains (eat them as a vegetable with a little sunflower oil, chives and mint). Add freshly squeezed lemon, grape or orange juice and a touch of honey to your barley water and drink at least two glasses a day.

I found plain barley water with a squeeze of lemon in it and a pinch of seasalt was a wonderfully refreshing pre-dinner drink when I was pregnant. When drunk at intervals during the hottest days of summer, I hardly felt the heat. Remember this for your baby too, because barley water is mild and bland and cleansing. My own children grew up on it and I am sure that this had something to do with their strong bones and perfect teeth.

Basil (Ocimum basilicum)

One or two basil leaves in 250 ml boiling water, sipped frequently, will do much to relieve morning sickness, nausea, vomiting and headaches. Chew a small leaf to help indigestion. Add a little basil to the daily salad – it has a tonic and carminative effect. A tip is to steep the flower whorls in salad oil and in salad vinegar to give the full taste and benefit of this remarkable herb.

Borage (Borago officinalis)
This is a wonderful, strengthening herb. It helps the kidneys manufacture cortisone by stimulating the adrenal cortex. Chopped fresh borage (10 ml) can be eaten daily to help constipation as it is mildly laxative. It will also greatly increase the milk flow for breastfeeding mums. A standard brew borage tea makes an excellent tonic all through your pregnancy and will keep the digestion smooth.

Aloe vera (Aloe barbadensis)
This common succulent rockery plant contains an incredibly soothing jelly that will quickly heal cuts, bites, grazes, scrapes, sunburn, rashes, stings, blisters, fever blisters or cold sores. It makes an excellent pot plant, too – all it requires is sunlight. Keep it growing near at hand for those everyday domestic mishaps. Simply break off a piece of the leaf and rub on the jelly. Apply frequently until the area is soothed. This is the best 'first aid' plant I know.

Cabbage (Brassica oleracea)
Warmed cabbage leaves for engorged, painful breasts are an ancient treatment, and in some country hospitals they are still used today in the maternity ward. Wear them inside your brassiere. Cabbage leaves ease milk flow, obstructions and keep the ducts open. This remedy works quickly and comfortingly.

Caraway (Carum carvi)
A tea made from 2 ml seeds in 250 ml boiling water is an excellent digestive. You can also add caraway tea to your baby's fruit juice for colic. It expels wind in both you and your baby, and it tones the liver and sweetens the bowels. If you give a teaspoon of caraway tea to your baby before meals, you will find he has hardly any wind or colic. If you suffer from heartburn, chew a few seeds or sip caraway tea, particularly if

the meal has been heavy and you are feeling uncomfortable.

Chopped fresh caraway leaves are delicious in salads. If you have a patch of garden or a window-box, caraway is easy to grow.

Carrots (Daucus carota)
Surprisingly, carrots are very important in both the antenatal and post-natal diet as well as in your baby's diet, which is why I make a special note of it here. Carrot juice, freshly extracted in a food processor, is a remarkable 'wonder food'. Just 2 ml every day will do much to prevent anaemia and jaundice. Mothers who eat raw grated carrots daily and drink carrot juice throughout their pregnancies hardly ever have jaundice in their newborn babies. Carrots are good for kidney and bladder ailments, muscle tone, building up resistance to infection, worms, varicose veins and improving eyesight.

Our grandmothers actually taught us this!

Catnip (Nepeta cataria)
This is a calming herb. Make a standard brew tea to soothe hiccoughs, heartburn, anxiety and tension in both you and your baby. As it is a refrigerant herb, it calms and cools and can be given to fretful and bedwetting children. Drink it as a nightcap too for pain relief, spasms in colic, and jangled nerves.

For baby, 2 ml before, during and after meals will ease colic. The same standard brew will also help regulate menstruation.

Cayenne pepper (Capsicum annuum)
Use cayenne pepper in cooking, but not only as a condiment. It is an antispasmodic and also brings down a fever. It can help to expel worms and is an effective intestinal cleanser. A pinch of cayenne sprinkled into a little hot water will help ease heartburn. Sip it slowly.

In fact, cayenne should ideally replace black and white pepper in the diet anyway!

Celery (Apium graveolens)
Fresh and green, chopped into the daily salad, celery is an important blood and kidney cleansing herb. It is also excellent if you are anaemic. A standard brew tea will bring down high blood pressure, steady the nerves (and, incidentally, improve eyesight). Use the seeds as a flavouring and include stems and leaves in soups, salads and stews.

Chamomile (Anthemis recutita)
Probably the most loved calming herb for babies – and for insomnia in adults! Chamomile is tonic and soothing and is recognised by the medical profession as a treatment for nervous, highly strung children. A standard brew tea is a good night time drink for expectant mothers. It will help increase milk flow and induce a good night's sleep once the baby is there. For children, use diluted with warm water and sweeten with honey. For babies, give 5 ml of the standard brew frequently to calm them down.

Comfrey (Symphytum officinale)
Comfrey is a healing herb – I believe it helps almost every ill mankind is prone to! Cook the leaves and eat as a spinach, or mince fresh leaves and add to salads. Make a standard brew tea for an excellent tonic for expectant mothers. I find it pleasant with a little lemon juice and honey added. Mince or grate 12,5 ml fresh leaves and add to 25-75 ml warm milk just before going to bed. During my own pregnancies I found this helped me sleep peacefully.

Coriander (Coriandrum sativum)
Coriander is an easy-to-grow herb and very attractive in all forms. The seeds and/or the leaves can be made into a tea (standard brew) to ease indigestion, nausea, flatulence and – for baby – colic. This brew is also a heart and stomach tonic and traditionally the remedy was used through the ages to 'ease the pain of childbirth'.

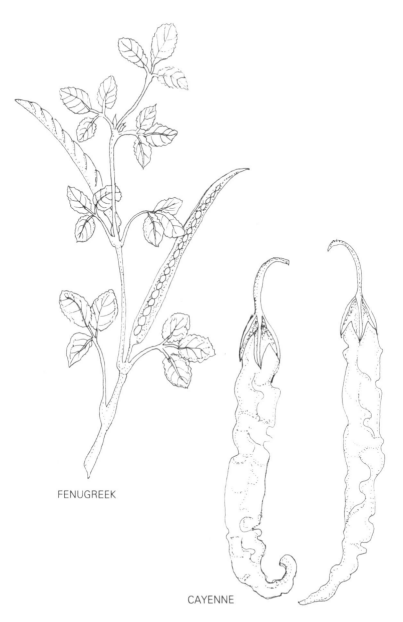

FENUGREEK

CAYENNE

27

For colicky babies, give 5-15 ml standard brew before meals and 5 ml after meals. Include a leaf or two in the daily salad to help indigestion. The following magical digestive medicine can be kept in the medicine chest and used by the whole family: Mix 125 ml crushed coriander seeds (roughly crush them in a pestle and mortar) into 125 ml honey. Place in a bottle and keep well sealed. Gently chew 2 ml of this mixture just before a meal or directly after a rich meal. Alternatively, mix 5 ml into 250 ml boiling water and sip slowly. For fretfulness or colic, give your baby 5 ml just before bedtime – it may ensure a peaceful night!

Dandelion (Taraxacum officinalis)
Dandelion leaves, far from being just a common garden weed, are filled with vitamins and minerals and they are so full of goodness that I include them here for both mother and child. Dandelion is blood cleansing, a blood tonic, an energiser, a muscle toner, and is superb for strengthening the walls of the arteries and veins. If it is included regularly in the diet, it will strengthen tooth enamel, so remember to give it to your children. It is also excellent for the treatment of jaundice and will aid diabetes and curb over-sleepiness. Try growing this common weed in a pot, ready for picking, at your kitchen door.

Dill (Antheum graveolens)
Probably the best known carminative for babies, dill is an ingredient in the famous gripe water we all know so well. It brings up wind and it is also rich in vitamins and minerals. For relief of indigestion and flatulence, make your own dill water:

In a screw-top bottle put 12,5 ml dill seeds (and a fresh leaf if you have one). Pour over 250 ml boiling water and add 10 ml apple cider vinegar and 12,5 ml honey. Shake well and keep in the fridge. Every time you need it warm a little before dosing the baby. Give 5-15 ml before meals, and 5 ml after meals.

Another 5 ml in the middle of the night will calm a fretting baby.

Add dill leaves and a few seeds to salads, stews and soups, if you have digestive upsets. This will reduce the likelihood of colic in your baby if you are breastfeeding and you will find your milk flow will increase. A standard brew tea is very soothing last thing at night; it will warm and relax you.

Elder (Sambucus nigra)

Elderflower tea (standard brew) makes a wonderful skin and hair treatment all through your pregnancy. A stronger brew – 500 ml flowers to 2 ℓ boiling water – can be used in your bath and as a rinse for face and hair.

Elder leaves can be used as a lotion for baby's rash or eczema: use 500 ml leaves boiled up in 2 ℓ water. Store excess in the fridge and warm a little every time you use it on the baby's skin.

Ripe elderberries, pounded in honey, make a soothing treatment for coughs and sore throats.

Fennel (Foeniculum officinale)

Fennel makes another wonderfully soothing tea, particularly effective for water retention. The leaves in the daily salad will relieve constipation and cramps. Fennel is another herb that aids the digestion and soothes colic and flatulence. Make a standard brew and give your baby 5 ml before a meal; it will help him digest it more easily. During pregnancy, chew a few fennel seeds to ease heartburn.

Fenugreek (Trigonella foenum-graecum)

The seed is the important part of this easily grown annual. It can be made into a rich, strength-giving tea, full of minerals, and will give tone and vitality to the muscles during pregnancy. It will also increase the flow of milk for breastfeeding mums. Take only 5 ml seeds and pour over 250 ml boiling water. Stand and steep. Add honey and lemon juice to taste, if desired. Drink when pleasantly warm. The tea can also be used to bring down a fever as it is cooling and soothing.

Feverfew (Chrysanthemum parthenium)
Feverfew is a traditional 'woman's herb'. A standard brew tea of this herb is said to help prevent a miscarriage, to help in a difficult labour and in the retention of the afterbirth. Feverfew is also both tonic and refreshing, but it is also extremely bitter, so sweeten with honey and add lemon juice. It will soothe a tension headache – eat a leaf with bread and butter. A poultice made from the crushed, pulped herb will do much to relieve painful piles.

Ginger (Zingiber officinale)
The properties of ginger are stimulating, warming, digestive and energising. Thinly slice a piece of fresh root (about the size of a 10c piece), pour boiling water over it, and stand for three minutes. As a drink it will greatly relieve neausea and morning sickness, indigestion, diarrhoea and headaches. It will also stimulate the menstrual cycle after childbirth and will combat exhaustion before and following the birth.
If you are travelling somewhere when pregnant, take along some glacé or candied ginger and nibble it to soothe nausea. A pinch of powdered ginger added to a cup of hot water is soothing too. The same brew will also ease labour pains.

Ground ivy (Glechoma hederacea)
This is a fragrant creeping hot-house plant, often grown in hanging baskets. It is a general tonic when made into a tea (standard brew) and it is used for retention of the afterbirth. As a tonic take 12,5 ml three times a day; for retention of afterbirth, the dose is 250 ml every two hours.

Hollyhock (Althaea rosea)
A standard brew tea made from hollyhock leaves will ease inflammation of the uterus, threatened miscarriage and

vaginitus. Bedouins apparently warm the leaves in wine and give them to expectant mothers to ward off a threatened miscarriage.

Any leftover tea can be added to the bath to soothe inflamed skin, fever or the rash on a baby's bottom. Cool, it can also be dabbed directly onto a rash or sunburn.

Honeysuckle (Lonicera species)
Honeysuckle tea (standard brew, using the flowers only) is a wonderful pick-me-up for those baby blues. Take a cup a day to lift depression.

Lavender (Lavandula spica, L. angustifolia)
Lavender tea is especially soothing. It will ease headaches, nausea and vomiting, so use it if you suffer from morning sickness. It makes a refreshing mouthwash too and can also be added to the bathwater. Try fresh lavender leaves and flowers tied in a facecloth or bath glove and used as a scrub for a relaxing, deeply cleansing bath when those trying early days with your newborn are getting you down. For a fretful, crying baby a teaspoon or two of lavender tea will help to soothe and calm.

Lemon (Citrus limonum)
Lemons are useful for bringing down fevers, cleansing the blood and soothing diarrhoea. As a tonic tea first thing in the morning for pregnant women one squeezed half of a medium sized lemon in 250 ml hot water will set you up for the day. The same tea, sipped hot or cold, will quickly relieve morning sickness or nausea. I found that even sucking a piece of lemon rind helped quell my morning sickness. Use the squeezed lemon for a quick beauty treatment on heels, elbows and nails.

Lucerne (Medicago sativa)
Also known as alfalfa, this is a most nourishing plant as it is rich in essential vitamins and minerals and is strengthening

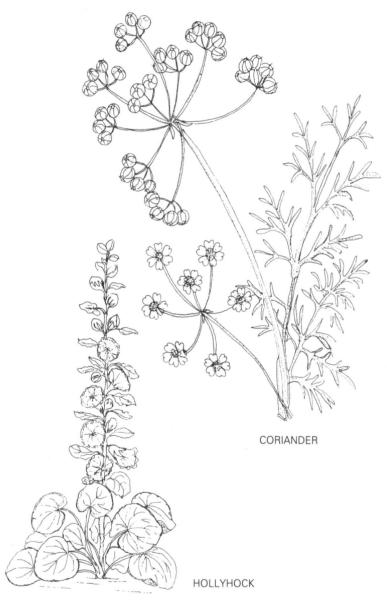

CORIANDER

HOLLYHOCK

and alkalising to the whole system. Lucerne can be sprouted and eaten in salads, but it is also an easy plant to grow in the garden. I cut my plants back frequently to ensure a crop of young shoots which I then add to salads, soups and stews, or make into teas. Lucerne is excellent for bladder and kidney ailments and for muscle tone and strength. If you take a cup of alfalfa tea daily in the last few weeks before your baby is due, this will improve your chances of an easy labour as your muscles will be well toned and strong.

Maidenhair fern (Adiantum capillus-veneris)
Maidenhair fern is a well-known hair tonic. Make a standard brew tea and use as a rinse to put shine and condition back into lifeless hair after the birth of your baby. It will also stimulate hair growth. A standard brew tea is good for chest colds, coughs and loosening a tight chest.

Marjoram (Origanum vulgare)
This is a digestive herb that works effectively on the whole system. A standard brew tea will soothe an acid stomach, morning sickness, nerves and fear. In nervous children it will also help dispel nightmares and prevent bedwetting (combine with catnip for the latter). Fresh marjoram as a flavouring for savoury dishes eliminates the need for salt and pepper – particularly helpful if you are on a salt-free diet. Warmed marjoram placed behind a baby's ears will soothe earache.

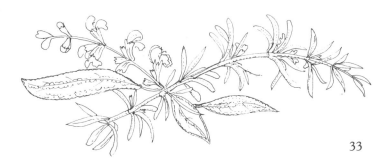

Melissa (Lemon balm, Melissa officinalis)

A much loved, calming herb, melissa is good for exhaustion, anxiety, nightmares, fears and nervousness. It is safe for children and extremely effective. It will quickly calm and soothe a restless baby: give 10 ml standard brew every half an hour. It will also stimulate expulsion of the afterbirth or delayed menstruation after the birth. It will bring down a fever and soothe gripes, colic and uterine disorders. Fresh leaves can be chopped up and included in salads. Tie a bunch of leaves in a muslin bag and put in the bath to calm hyperactive children. Alternatively, add 125 ml standard brew to 125 ml juice.

Mint (Mentha species)

Mint quells stomach pains and gas. It is a digestive aid as it combats acidity and heartburn. Chew a mint leaf for immediate relief if heartburn is a problem in your pregnancy. A standard brew tea will settle nausea and morning sickness and will also ease suppressed urine and menstruation. For a bad headache, soak a few slices of raw potato in a strong mint tea, then apply them to the forehead, holding them in place with a cloth which has been wrung out in the tea.

Diarrhoea, vomiting, gastritis and dysentery all respond to mint tea. There are many varieties, but peppermint is probably the best known and the most used. Peppermint tea makes an excellent nightcap for tired or depressed mums. It will also ease constipation and painful menstruation.

Nettle (Urtica dioica)

There are few plants that contain as much in the way of minerals, vitamins and chlorophyll as the nettle. The formic acid on the nettle's fine hairs is responsible for its sting – so wear gloves when you pick the leaves. For the expectant mother, nettle spinach or nettle soup is surprisingly delicious and can do much to tone and strengthen the blood vessels, expel mucus from the body and combat anaemia. Nettle also aids expulsion of kidney stones. As a standard brew tea it will act as a tonic, keeping you fit and free from infection.

Oats (Avena sativum)
Oats should form an important part of the diet during pregnancy and after the birth of the baby. It is, in fact, one food that can be taken when nothing else can be tolerated. It is a nerve and blood tonic and will help build strong teeth, hair and nails. It is rich in the B vitamins, low in starch and high in mineral content. It is also an effective anti-depressant: if you suffer from the post-natal blues, use oats in a thin gruel or tea, sipped with honey. Alternatively, eat as a porridge with milk and honey, or uncooked in muesli with fresh fruit and yoghurt. Look for the non-instant oats (avoid all instant foods during pregnancy) in health food shops and in some supermarkets.

Parsley (Petroselinum crispum)
Parsley tea has a beneficial effect on the urinary system and is an excellent treatment for kidney and bladder complaints. Warmed, bruised leaves packed into the brassiere will ease swollen, painful breasts. When trying to wean your baby, this will also help dry up your milk.

Pennyroyal (Mentha pulegium)
NB Pennyroyal tea should not be taken when you are pregnant. It is only an after-care tea.

For suppressed menstruation, 125 ml hot pennyroyal tea (standard brew) taken after a hot bath at night, and the same amount taken morning and evening, will restore energy to an exhausted mother after childbirth.

Periwinkle (Vinca major)
Make a standard brew tea and take 12,5 ml three times a day,

sweetened with honey, for calming the nerves. Use the rest of the tea, warmed, as a compress around the breasts to help dry up excess milk and excessive dripping from the nipples. Leave on for an hour. Repeat three to four times during the day.

Pineapple (Ananas comosus)
Pineapple is filled with vitamins and minerals and fresh slices of pineapple should be part of your diet throughout pregnancy. Pineapple juice is also an excellent diuretic and helps ease water retention. It will help bring down urine after the birth of the baby.

Plantain (Plantago major)
This common weed has soothing qualities. A standard brew tea can be used as an external poultice for piles (haemorrhoids). Alternatively, crush the leaves and apply directly to the area.

Raspberry (Rubus idaeus)
Traditionally considered to prevent miscarriage and to tone the muscles, raspberry is a safe, effective herb for pregnant women. A standard brew tea, taken frequently throughout the day, is pleasant and refreshing and works deeply within the muscles and uterus. Sweeten with honey if desired.

Try to use fresh raspberry leaves; they grow easily in most places but do not bear fruit in the hotter areas. They multiply by suckers and two or three plants will produce a good crop of leaves. Once you have them in your garden, they will be there to stay. The leaf contains an active principle called fragrine, which acts particularly on the female reproductive organs, the muscles of the pelvis and uterus. As a tea it is an excellent tonic throughout pregnancy and during labour and will also help bring down the afterbirth. Raspberry leaf tea will bring relief from morning sickness. It can be used to treat diarrhoea and dysentery and bring down a fever in a small baby. It will also strengthen a prolapsed uterus. As a pick-me-up after the

36

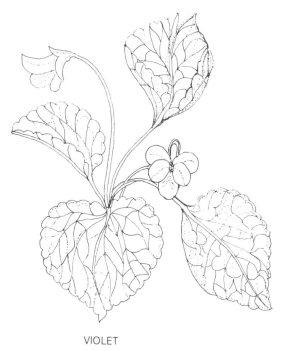

VIOLET

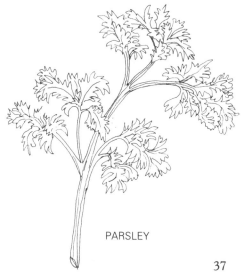

PARSLEY

37

birth of your baby drink raspberry tea to combat anaemia, fatigue and lack of energy. It will also put some colour back into your cheeks!

Rose

Rose petals are both soothing and calming, and the essential oil of roses has been used for hundreds of years as a heart and brain tonic, as well as a tonic for the uterus and ovaries. The petals can be used to make a tea (standard brew), syrup or jam to calm the nerves. (I use the deeply scented red rose 'Crimson Glory'.) The tea is also beneficial for a threatened miscarriage and for strengthening the heart before the birth of the baby.

Rose petals in the bath or eaten in a salad are not only good for the skin, but are gently astringent too. Try pounding 250 ml honey and a cup of petals together. Spread a little of the mixture on a slice of bread or take approximately 5-10 ml in hot water every day.

Rosemary (Rosmarinus officinalis)

Rosemary is a remarkable herb: it is used to treat high blood pressure, heart ailments, headaches, threatened miscarriage and nervous ailments. Used externally, rosemary tea will revitalise and stimulate dull hair after your baby is born, and will also check falling, damaged hair. If you are tired and listless, a standard brew tea is wonderful first thing in the morning.

Rue (Ruta graveolens)

Pungent and powerful rue is a much respected herb in herbal medicine. It is potent and bitter and the dosage is only 5 ml of fresh leaves to 500 ml boiling water, prepared as for a standard brew. Take 25 ml morning and evening for heart and nervous ailments, and also for congestion of the uterus and pains in pregnancy. A little warmed brew, sweetened with honey (10 ml brew to 2 ml honey) is good for colic in babies.

A stock remedy that has been used for hundreds of years to remove worms from children is worth trying: just insert an oiled sprig of rue into the anus at night.

Sage (Salvia officinalis)
A much loved herb, sage is probably known best for its soothing properties in treating coughs, colds and fevers. The standard brew tea, however, is also good for nervousness, digestive discomfort, flatulence and constipation. It will increase the milk yield in breastfeeding mothers and give tonic properties to the milk.

Salad burnet (Sanguisorba officinalis)
This is a tonic herb and, as a tea, will cleanse blood disorders and skin problems. Use as a wash on the skin or add to the bathwater. It is soothing and gentle for sunburnt skin and can be used as a wash for baby's eczema or nappy rash.

Southernwood (Artemisia abrotanum)
This is a renowned 'female' herb and is excellent for treating bladder or kidney problems: make a standard brew and take 125 ml morning and evening. It also makes a good wash and lotion for baby's rashes and scalp infections: use 5-20 ml two to three times a day. (Because it is not very palatable, it is perhaps best used as a wash.)

Strawberry (Fragaria vesca)
Strawberries are an effective treatment for blood disorders and the fruit is excellent for anaemia, lowered vitality and as a nerve tonic. When the fruit is not in season a standard brew tea of the leaves can be used for bowel disorders, fevers, irregular menstruation and to prevent miscarriage. It will also clear liver disorders and excessive perspiration. Externally, it can be used on the skin for rashes and eczema, and as a lotion for sore eyes and styes.

Sweetcorn (Zea mays)
Sweetcorn should be an essential part of our diet. To use young sweetcorn at their best, strip off their cobs and toss them in a salad. The silk found in the husk is a safe treatment for kidney and bladder ailments; it will also help prevent bedwetting in children. Use some chopped raw silk in salads or make a standard brew tea. Drink 125 ml three times a day or, for babies, give 10 ml twice a day.

Thyme (Thymus vulgaris, T. serpyllum)
These thymes and the lemon flavoured thyme (*Thymus citriodorus*) are natural antiseptics. Thyme soothes indigestion, flatulence, nervousness, liver ailments, headaches and even nightmares. It helps expel the afterbirth and is excellent in the treatment of an inflamed or diseased uterus. It can also give relief in cases of engorged breasts.

Vine (Vitis vinifera)
Grapevine leaves, tendrils and grapes are so beneficial to all round health that for expectant mothers they act as a tonic for the whole system. Young leaves and tendrils can be made into a health-giving tea (standard brew) to bring down a fever, relieve constipation, lift depression and tone the blood.

Watercress (Nasturtium officinale)
Watercress is an effective treatment for blood disorders. For mothers having difficulty breastfeeding, it will increase the milk flow; chop up 125 ml watercress, steep in a cup of slightly warmed milk. Allow the milk to cool and, when cold, drink the liquid (eat the watercress afterwards). You will find your milk flow increases quickly. Watercress also helps ease a stiff back and stiff joints.

Yarrow (Achillea millefolium)
A warmed yarrow leaf compress will soothe painful haemorrhoids. Apply externally.

Preparing for the birth

Pamper yourself in the last month before your baby is born. It is the last chance in a long while you will get to do so. These last few weeks are most important for both you and your baby. Try to enjoy each day and live every moment to the full. Life will never be the same again!

Keep an eye on the following checklist:

- *Sleep* Be sure to get as much as you can. Rest in the afternoons if at all possible. If you have other children, try to farm them out to friends for a couple of hours. Read and relax all you can. Go to bed early. You need to build up strength for the sleepless days and nights ahead.

- *Avoid watching TV* Television 'rays' are still an unknown quantity. Tests are being done but no one is yet quite sure of the effect they have on human life. Avoid, therefore, exposing your unborn child to any rays, X-rays, laser beams, microwaves, computer rays, electric blanket, etc.

- *Fluids* In this last month fluid intake is tremendously important. Drink fresh fruit juice, plenty of water, and calming herb teas. Increase your intake of fresh milk.

- *Diet* What you eat in these vital weeks is of utmost importance. Your baby is big now and he or she will be needing extra food in preparation for entering into the world.

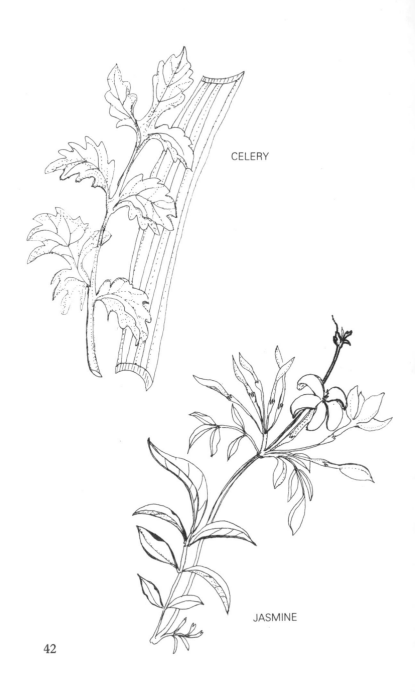

CELERY

JASMINE

Increase your intake of vitamins E and C. Pantothenic acid found in the B vitamins taken just before the birth helps combat stress. Make sure to eat plain yoghurt daily, and lots of green leafy vegetables, in the last week especially, to provide vitamin K (which prevents haemorrhaging). Step up calcium intake: remember that dolomite acts as a pain-killer and may be helpful if you are in any discomfort. In general try to eat only *whole* foods and avoid junk foods or drinks during this period.

● *Exercise* Step up your exercise routine to keep your body tuned and supple in preparation for labour. Do exercises every day under the supervision of or taking the advice of your physiotherapist or antenatal instructor. Walk some-where every day, even if it is only to the corner shop.

● *Nipple treatment* Massage cream into your nipples to strengthen them before your baby begins breastfeeding. Cracked nipples is a common but avoidable problem when you first start feeding and, if left untreated, can be very sore indeed.

● *Stretchmark massage* As the baby grows very quickly in this last month, do not neglect this important task.

● *Be happy* Read, listen to peaceful music, avoid all stressful people, places and occasions if you possibly can.

● *Deep breathing* Concentrate on your breathing exercises; allow them to become automatic to you. You will probably be feeling fairly uncomfortable now and anxious for the baby to be born.

● *Case packed* Don't be caught unawares – have your case ready at least six weeks before you are due. Prepare the baby's room a month in advance, and anything else in the home that needs doing, so that this last month is a holiday.

A day or two before you are due, wash your hair, do your nails and have a friend do your feet, pedicure and massage – you will not be able to reach them, and you won't have time once the baby is there. Above all, be happy. You are about to become a mother!

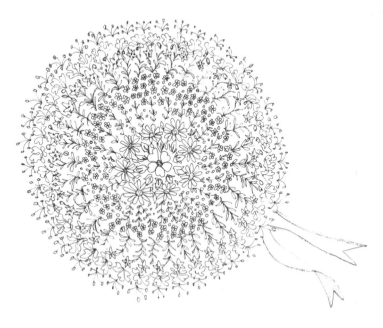

The newborn

The first few weeks after your baby is born can be a confusing, often exhausting time, especially for first-time mothers. 'Nobody told me it would be like this!' and 'I never knew it was possible to be so tired!' are perhaps the two refrains heard most often from new mothers. Above all try to relax until you find your routine. An unstressed mother goes a long way to making an unstressed baby. Now is the time when you will lay the foundation for your relationship with your new son or daughter. It is the time for bonding and nurturing, for intimacy and loving closeness.

BREASTFEEDING

This is the greatest gift you can give to your child. If it is at all possible, I urge you to breastfeed. The sucking reflex in a newborn baby is very strong and the infant should be put to the breast as soon as possible. The first 'food' your baby will get from sucking is called 'colostrum'. This watery substance is rich in protein and will prevent him or her falling prey to infection in these first few days. While sucking is instinctive and comforting to your baby, it also stimulates the breasts into releasing the milk.

If you have looked after yourself throughout your pregnancy, you should have no difficulty breastfeeding. Do not worry that your baby is not getting enough milk; he will take what he needs and your breasts will respond accordingly. Every baby's needs are different and you will find what suits your child best as the weeks go by. You will learn to recognise a 'hungry' cry and will probably have a more contented baby if you 'demand feed'. In other words do not try to stick to a rigid

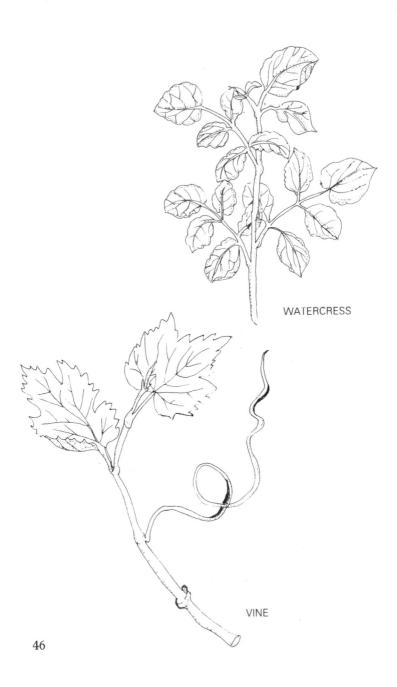

WATERCRESS

VINE

46

four hourly schedule. If your baby seems hungry every two or three hours, feed him. He will soon settle into a routine.

Breastfeeding is the easiest and best way of feeding your baby: he gets the perfectly balanced food served at the perfect temperature. It is the opportunity for him to get to know your smell and your touch and respond to it as to no other. Breast-feeding bonds you and your baby for all time.

Your diet while breastfeeding

Make sure that you keep up your fluid intake – fresh milk, water, bland fruit juices (avoid undiluted orange juice for a few weeks) and herb teas. You will need now to add more Brewer's yeast to your diet; the powdered form is excellent. Increase your intake of liver, wheatgerm, kelp and extra protein. Keep up your vitamins. Keep a 'nibble-bowl' handy and fill it with raisins, almonds and sunflower seeds.

The following is an energy-giving recipe for mums who are breastfeeding.

NURSING MOTHER'S ENERGISER

500 ml whole milk
125 ml non-instant powdered milk
12,5 ml debittered Brewer's yeast
12,5 ml sunflower oil
125 ml mashed fruit (eg banana, grapes, peach, pawpaw)
1 egg
3 bonemeal tablets, crushed
10 ml fresh mint, chopped (melissa or sage are also good)
12,5 ml lecithin granules

Whirl all ingredients in a blender. Add another 500 ml milk. Drink 60-125 ml at intervals throughout the day (you should have finished it by bedtime). Increase yeast after a week or two up to 37,5 ml.

Herbs to help milk flow

Borage, dill, fenugreek, raspberry, and periwinkle are all good for keeping up your milk flow. The last mentioned will also help dry up dripping breasts. Lettuce cooked in milk will increase milk flow and also help you sleep: Boil up one chopped lettuce in 1 ℓ milk (use the dark outer leaves as well). Simmer for 5 minutes with the lid half on. Drain and use the milk as a drink, storing excess in the fridge to add to soup. Eat the leaves with a little chopped celery and thyme as a vegetable. It is surprisingly delicious.

Cracked nipples/Engorged breasts

If you have taken proper care to harden your nipples during your pregnancy in preparation for breastfeeding, cracked nipples should not be a problem. If you feel a sharp, shooting pain in your nipple when the baby is feeding, it is probably a cracked nipple. This is a painful condition and should be treated quickly. Immediately stop feeding on that side and express your milk manually or with a breast pump. Do not be tempted to put on baby oil; rather use a vitamin E and comfrey cream, or dab on Friar's Balsam with cotton wool. Make sure that you wash well before nursing again.

Parsley packed into the brassiere or warmed cabbage leaves will ease a blocked duct or painful, engorged breasts. Thyme works well this way too, as does the inner side of a pawpaw skin.

For how long should you breastfeed?

You should try to breastfeed for at least three months to give your baby a good start in building up resistance to infection and getting the quality and quantity of nourishment he needs. If it is possible to continue for longer, then do keep it up for as long as your baby wants to. Your baby will indicate when he is losing interest in the breast (probably round about 8 to 9 months). My first two children were big babies and needed extra food by six months. I started then to supplement their diets with cow's milk and solids. The youngest one was contented to nurse until she was eight months old.

FORMULA FEEDING

If you are unable to breastfeed for any reason (eg if you have to return to work or if you are separated from your baby), you can prepare your own bottle feeds. Never allow a small baby to feed by himself propped up on a pillow. Firstly it is dangerous – a baby can easily choke; secondly, your baby needs to be cuddled and held and talked to while feeding. Give yourself this time with him and let him know that he is loved. The following milk formula is safe after six months if a proprietary tinned one is not available. It is an old-fashioned one and I have used it most successfully. However, you should always ask the advice of your doctor or clinic sister first.

Start by adding one-third boiled cow's milk to two-thirds boiled water for one week. Increase to half boiled water and half boiled milk the second week. In the third week mix two-thirds milk to one-third water and finally go on to full strength cow's milk by the fourth week. Pour the formula into sterilised bottles and keep in the fridge. I found this an excellent way of adding more substance to feeds and eventually replaced the midday breastfeed with this bottle. Let the baby take all he needs and do not force him. He will adjust at his own speed.

Sterilising

Once you switch to formula or supplementary feeding, you will need to sterilise bottles, teats and formula. The easiest way of doing this is to make up the day's formula early by filling three, four or five bottles, covering with teats and

49

placing them all in a steamer or large pot with a rack on which they can stand, covering with a lid. The boiling water and steam sterilises the bottles and no valuable protein is lost in the process.

Keep the bottles in the fridge and, when required, take a bottle and stand it in a jug of hot water until it is the required temperature (lukewarm).

Remember that babies get thirsty as well as hungry. A sterilised bottle with plain boiled water in it should always be on hand. Should you have a colicky baby, add a little herb tea (standard brew) to the water: mint, melissa, dill, fennel and caraway are all perfectly safe and very soothing.

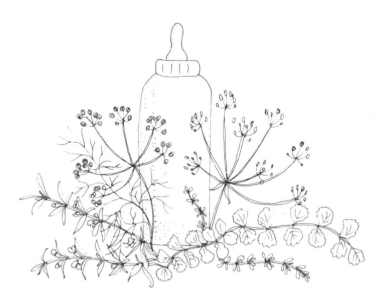

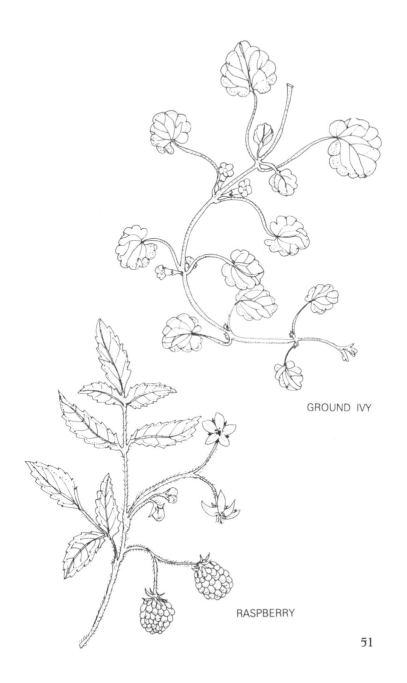

GROUND IVY

RASPBERRY

51

The older baby

As he grows older your baby will require more fluids. Fruit juices, freshly squeezed and diluted, can now be added to his diet. Add a little mint or catnip tea if the fruit is a little acid. If you think it may be too sour, put in 2-5 ml honey. Beware of adding sweeteners to his diet at this early stage. Try not to encourage a sweet tooth. The only acceptable sweetener is honey, and then it must be used sparingly.

INTRODUCING SOLIDS

Once your baby has indicated that his breast or formula feeds no longer satisfy his hunger completely, it is time to introduce solids. Some babies require solids sooner than others, but his milk feeds should be enough until he is three months old. Be guided by your doctor or clinic sister.

The first and easiest solid should be in the form of porridge at breakfast time. Oatmeal porridge is a nourishing starter. Do not use instant oats; find the real, large-flake kind obtainable from health food shops and some supermarkets. Make it rather runny and press it through a sieve with a wooden spoon, or liquidise it. Mix in a little boiled milk or plain yoghurt and a touch of honey.

STEAMED VEGETABLES AND FRUIT

You will soon find your baby is ready for a good lunch. Invest in a steamer if you do not already have one. Boiling vegetables and fruit reduces their nutritional value and allows precious vitamins and minerals to escape. A steamer, particularly one with two or three layers, works well and allows you to do both fruit and vegetables at the same time.

Suitable vegetables to start off with are: squash, courgettes, peas, green beans, carrots, pumpkin, beetroot, cabbage, spinach, lettuce, cauliflower, broccoli, sweet potatoes and potatoes. All of these can be steamed – lettuce too – and then put through a liquidiser with a little of the water, or pressed through a sieve with a wooden spoon.

Serve plain vegetables to start with, and introduce one different flavour at a time. Give your baby three or four teaspoons for lunch and gradually increase the amount to two or three tablespoons. He will also let you know when he has had enough. As he gets used to new tastes and textures, add in some chicken jelly, or the water in which chicken was boiled. Try putting in half a teaspoon of Marmite; some babies enjoy the change of taste and the saltiness.

Suitable fruits to start off with are: apples, peaches and pears. These three are the most suitable for steaming. Pawpaw, grapes (peeled and pipped), mangos and overripe bananas can also be given early on, but are best served raw, mashed and sieved.

Always introduce one new taste at a time to see if your baby likes it; he will let you know in no uncertain terms if he doesn't! Resist sweetening food with sugar; always try to keep food as natural as possible. Add a little plain yoghurt by way of a change, or some chunky cottage cheese.

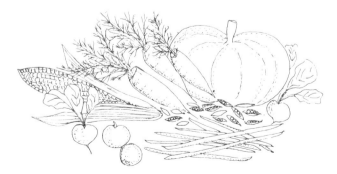

PROTEIN

Meat, chicken and fish are the best sources of protein and can be gradually added to the diet after three months. Prepare by steaming or boiling as this is the most easily digestible method for the baby.

Boiled chicken

Place one chicken piece (eg breast) in a pot with enough water to cover. Add a stick of celery, one thumb-length sprig of thyme, a squeeze of lemon juice and 5 ml iodised seasalt. Cover and simmer for approximately an hour or until chicken is tender.

Drain and save the water and keep it in a sealed container in the fridge. Mix a spoon or two of this 'jelly' (it will set once in the fridge) with the baby's vegetables. Finely mince some of the chicken breast and mix it in with the vegetables. Offer a teaspoon at a time at the midday meal.

Beef or liver stew

Place diced beef or liver in a pot, add water (to which a little debittered yeast has been added) and add a squeeze of lemon juice, a pinch or two of seasalt, a sprig of marjoram or fennel, and a stick of celery. Boil up in enough water to just cover the chopped pieces. Mince finely when tender and add a teaspoon or two to baby's vegetables, with some of the gravy.

Steamed fish

Place a piece of deboned fish in a steamer. Squeeze over it a little lemon juice and 12,5 ml plain yoghurt. Add a pinch of seasalt. Steam until tender. Flake the fish and mix in with the baby's vegetables (just two to three teaspoons to start with). Spoon over a little yoghurt sauce. Never fry fish for a baby as it is very indigestible done this way. Fish is an important source of phosphorus and iodine and should be included in the diet at least once a week.

BASIC MENU UP TO SIX MONTHS

Milk is still the major item in the baby's diet up to six months. If your baby is also on solids, he should be getting porridge in the morning, with a little plain yoghurt added; and at midday, steamed fruit and vegetables, with protein from chicken, meat and fish.

In the beginning, as you start him off on solids, give him his milk first, then top up with solids. Later, once he is used to new tastes and textures, start the meal with solids and top up with milk.

It is a good idea to keep a notebook on his early eating patterns so that anything that may cause a rash or diarrhoea can be identified quickly and eliminated from the diet.

FROM SIX MONTHS TO ONE YEAR

Gradually introduce your baby to egg yolk (discard the white) by lightly boiling an egg, and mixing it into his porridge, a teaspoon of yolk at a time. You can also make a simple custard, using milk and egg and a touch of honey.

CUSTARD

375 ml milk
2-5 ml honey
2 egg yolks, beaten

Bring milk and honey to the boil in a double boiler, or on a very low heat. Add the egg yolks and keep stirring (it curdles easily – if it does, liquidise it), allowing it to thicken gently. If you want a thicker custard, stir 10 ml cornflour into a little cold milk and add to the mixture.

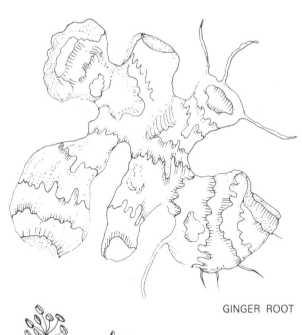

GINGER ROOT

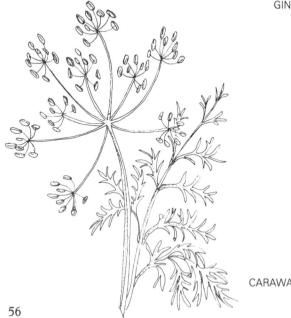

CARAWAY

56

If you leave out the honey, you can add a little of this custard to minced fish or chicken, or to mashed potatoes.

CURD CHEESE

This is full of nutrition and can be added to porridge, vegetables or fruit. As you will still be pureeing everything in a liquidiser or through a sieve, it will enrich whatever it is added to and the baby will accept the taste.

500 ml milk
1 sprig melissa or lemon thyme

Place herb in the milk and allow to stand overnight out of the fridge, keeping the container covered. Next day, when it is thick and sour, discard the herbs, and pour through a muslin cloth to let the whey drip out. Use the curd in mashed banana, sparingly to start with. My babies all loved it! Cover and keep excess in the fridge.

RIPE BANANAS

Only very ripe bananas should be used. Choose the brown, blotchy skinned ones that are soft to the touch.

AVOCADO

Mashed avocado is very easy to digest and rich in vitamins and minerals.

ORANGES

Choose very sweet ones, squeeze out the juice and add it to herb teas (eg melissa, standard brew), or peel and put them through a liquidiser and add to mashed pawpaw or banana.

YOGHURT

Yoghurt is more easily digested than milk, but be sure to use only plain yoghurt, never the coloured fruit ones.

SPROUTS

Mung beans and alfalfa can be sprouted easily and a few, liquidised, in the baby's porridge or vegetables, can be introduced now. Sprouts are highly nutritious; their protein, vitamin and mineral content surpasses most other foodstuffs. They should become part of your family's daily menu and, if given now, will give your baby a taste for this health food throughout his life.

RAW FOODS

From ten months onwards your baby can safely have minced or pureed raw foods: carrots, beetroot, apple, celery, cucumber and tomato are all suitable (Raw beetroot is excellent, but may colour his stools and urine pink – do not be alarmed.)

PULSES

Peas, beans, lentils, chickpeas and soya beans all need to be soaked overnight, then slowly cooked and pureed with water. I soak mine with a sprig of thyme, marjoram or a dill leaf, then cook them with fresh marjoram or thyme, and two to three fennel or dill leaves: these are all digestive aids. Mix a little of this pureed mush into vegetables. Mix with mashed avocado and yoghurt.

CHEESE

Cottage cheese is easily tolerated and can be mixed with steamed fruit; other mild cheeses can be introduced too by finely grating a little and stirring it into his vegetables. Do not cook cheese as this makes it indigestible.

NUTS AND SUNFLOWER SEEDS

Almonds or pecan nuts can be minced with sunflower seeds into a flour and added to fruit or vegetable dishes. Rich in protein and minerals, they are important in the baby's diet. Never give your baby peanuts.

CAROB

Chocolate is not suitable for babies (or for you!). Rather use carob from the carob pod, which is a more natural flavouring and contains vitamins A, D and B riboflavin and niacin – all important for glowing health.

POINTS TO REMEMBER

- *Sweetening* A sweet tooth is cultivated – not inherited! Keep sweetening to a minimum, and use only honey as an additive.

- *Colourants* These can cause allergies, so try to avoid them wherever possible.

- *Preservatives* Read the ingredients on every package you buy. Get to know what unnatural substances are in prepared foods and avoid them.

- Feed your baby only the best fresh, natural, uncontaminated food. Prepare it as naturally as possible, and as he grows older feed him as much raw food as possible. Grow your own, if at all feasible.

- Read up on health and nutrition; there are any number of

books on the subject available from your local library.

- Avoid fast foods, junk foods, sweets, crisps, icecream and refined foods. There are a vast number of substitutes for snack foods that are tasty and nutritious.

- Keep up intake of natural vitamins for both your baby and yourself.

TEETHING AND FINGER FOODS

After your baby has cut his first teeth, he will start putting everything into his mouth. Now is the time to provide him with chewable foods which will aid his teeth formation and soothe his gums.

RUSKS

These can give him lots of chewing fun. Make your own, cutting them large enough for him to handle without choking:

10 slices homemade wholewheat bread (about 2 cm thick)
180 ml hot water into which 15 ml yeast extract (eg Marmite) has been dissolved.

Cut the slices into fingers and, using a pastry brush, brush the yeast extract and water onto all sides of the bread. Space a little apart on a wire cake cooler and bake at 150 °C for about 1½ hours until crisp and dry. Cool and store in a tin.

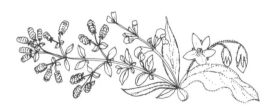

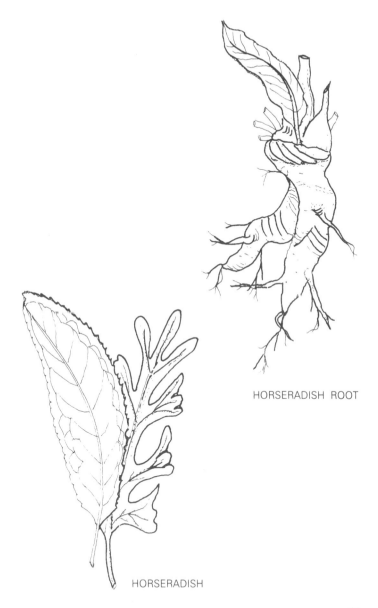

HORSERADISH ROOT

HORSERADISH

61

TEETHING BISCUITS

62,5 ml wholewheat flour
62,5 ml soy flour
18 ml soft honey
1 egg yolk
12,5 ml sunflower oil
10 ml mint or thyme, chopped
enough milk to make a stiff dough

Mix all ingredients together, slowly adding the milk last of all. Pinch off pieces of dough and roll into a 2 cm thick sausage about 8 cm long. Bake at 180° for about 20 minutes. When cool, store in an airtight tin.

CHOPPED FOODS

Gradually get your baby used to chopped or roughly mashed foods rather than purees. This will get him chewing which is good for teething too. Mix grated raw carrot or chopped tomatoes into his mashed food. Set out trays of *finger foods* for him to try. These are important in the baby's diet and, as he is intrigued by different objects now, and will pick up and put different things into his mouth, he will enjoy this activity. He will also search out the things that his system needs. I made notes on the selection of foods my babies liked from day to day and at the end of the week it balanced out surprisingly well. Finger foods will teach independence too and will get your children interested in food.

Set out manageable pieces of any of the following on a plate or tray, but never leave a baby to eat on his own in case he chokes. Let him experiment without you hovering, but keep an eye on him.

Hardboiled egg, sliced; tomato; green peas, cooked; cucumber; celery stick; banana; pear; carrot sticks; cubes of cheese; raisins; wholewheat bread made into tiny sandwiches with cottage cheese; small pieces of *boned* cooked fish, chicken or meat, or a small pile of cooked minced meat; few grapes, peeled and seeded; piece of peach, peeled; small pile of chopped sprouts.

BASIC MENU FOR TWELVE MONTHS AND UPWARDS

Your baby is now becoming a child. He is probably starting to take his first shaky steps and 'talking' to you non-stop. He is doubtless displaying a mind of his own too and, hopefully, if you have taken care over his diet, he is happy, healthy and sturdy. You can now broaden his diet considerably.

Breakfast: porridge, yoghurt (plain), little honey to sweeten. Boiled or scrambled egg. Wholewheat toast with yeast extract (eg Marmite) or touch of honey. Mug of milk to drink. Piece of fruit (eg pawpaw, peach etc).

Mid-morning: fresh fruit juice with herb tea. Rusk or biscuit.

Lunch: Steamed vegetables, meat, fish or chicken. Salad finger foods. Fresh fruit, custard. Mug of milk.

Afternoon snack: fresh fruit juice, fruit pieces.

Supper: soup, wholewheat bread, sandwich or savoury dish. Fruit (eg banana mashed with yoghurt or cottage cheese). Mug of milk.

Remember to season food with herbs rather than salt and pepper. A little coarse seasalt is acceptable.

Food for healthy kids

Remember that the correct, healthy way of eating learned as a baby will become a way of life as your children grow up. It will give them pride in their bodies and the way they look. Self-esteem and a feeling of self-worth are important fundamentals for a happy life. The following are a few recipes my own children have thrived on and enjoyed. Develop your own variations as you go along, and change them around to encourage an interest in mealtimes.

BREAKFAST STANDBY

In a thermos flask the night before, pour in 125 ml oats that have been mixed with 375 ml hot water. Add 12,5 ml seedless raisins, 12,5 ml almond meal ground in a coffee grinder, 12,5 ml sunflower seeds and 12,5 ml wheatgerm. Shake up well and seal.

Next morning the mixture will be fluffy and swollen up. Serve with a little warm milk and yoghurt and a touch of honey. My children grew to love this porridge, particularly on a winter morning, as it set them up for the day. They still enjoy it today!

HOMEMADE YOGHURT

Yoghurt, plain and unsweetened, is easy to make. It is a superb health food, and easily assimilated by the body. As all the family benefit from yoghurt, a good quantity should always be at hand. (I use it in baking as well as in porridge or muesli, and in sauces.)

500 ml whole milk
25 ml natural yoghurt
36,5 ml skim milk powder

Bring the milk to the boil and simmer for four or five minutes. Allow to cool to 43 °C, ie pleasantly warm. Mix the yoghurt and milk powder and pour in a little of the boiled milk, stirring well. Add the rest of the milk, stirring continually. If you have a yoghurt maker, pour the mixture into it; if you don't, pour it into a wide-necked thermos flask. The secret is to leave it undisturbed for about 5 hours or until it is set. (If you leave it in the thermos for too long it will taste too acid.) Once it is set – between 5-8 hours – place in the fridge and use as required.

YOGHURT RECIPES

Instead of adding milk, cream or custard to fruit or porridge, use plain yoghurt. The following flavourings will be great favourites with your baby as well as older children.

Sweet

● *Pureed fruit* (eg apples, strawberries, pawpaw, mango, peaches, bananas). Add a pinch of cinnamon and a little honey. Whirl in some plain yoghurt and serve as a dessert.

● Soak *dried peaches* or apple rings in water overnight. Chop or mince and add to yoghurt. Toss in a few chopped dates if you like.

● Put a tablespoon each of *almonds* and sunflower seeds

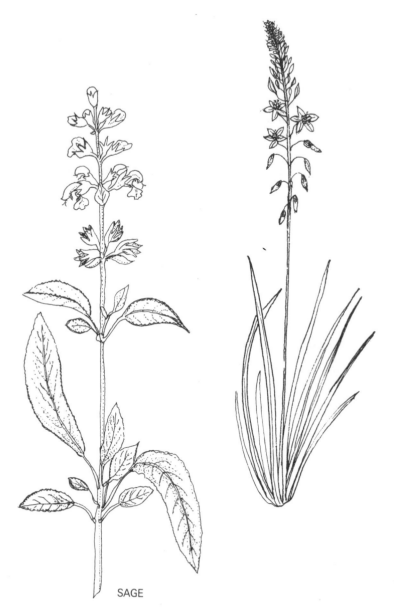

SAGE

through a wheatmill or coffee grinder. Mix into 125 ml yoghurt and add a touch of honey or molasses.

Savoury

- Liquidise a *peeled tomato* with two cucumber slices (also peeled) into 125 ml yoghurt. Serve as a soup.

- Add 25 ml finely chopped or minced raw *carrots*, celery and lettuce to 125 ml yoghurt. Mix well and serve as a vegetable.

- Add mild grated cheese and a little finely minced celery or spinach to yoghurt.

BANANA OATS

This is a delicious breakfast dish. The whole family will love it.

125 ml large-flake, non-instant oats (for baby, mill them)
200 ml milk
½ ripe banana, mashed
60 ml plain yoghurt

Cook oats gently in the milk, and blend in banana and yoghurt. Stir well into oats and cook one minute more. Serve with a touch of honey.

HEALTH SOUP (serves 6)

125 ml barley, soaked overnight in water
125 ml haricot, kidney or butter beans, soaked overnight in water
2 stalks celery, chopped
1 onion, chopped
2-3 tomatoes, skinned and chopped

2 carrots, grated
25 ml debittered yeast
250 ml chopped spinach or cabbage
250 ml chopped greens (eg borage, dandelion, comfrey etc)
seasalt
thyme or marjoram
lemon juice
oil
2 ℓ water or stock

Brown the onions and the celery in a little oil. Add all the other ingredients, cover and simmer until the beans and barley are tender. Adjust seasoning to taste. Liquidise a portion for the baby and serve it to him with fingers of buttered wholewheat toast. He will enjoy dipping the toast into the bowl. Soon he will enjoy the soup served unliquidised as he sees how the rest of the family eat it.

Vary this soup by adding a chicken carcass or soup bones, or stir in a cup or two of yoghurt. Use whatever vegetables are in season – courgettes, leeks, kohlrabi, cauliflower, broccoli and pumpkin all make delicious variations.

COLD SOUP (serves 6)

250 ml chopped celery
2 tomatoes, skinned and chopped
1 small lettuce, chopped
1 cucumber, chopped
2 carrots, grated
250-500 ml chopped greens (eg spinach, dandelion leaves, comfrey leaves, borage etc)
250 ml cooked beans, lentils or peas
thyme or marjoram
seasalt
lemon juice to taste
500-750 ml water or stock
500-750 ml yoghurt

Whirl all ingredients in a liquidiser. Sprinkle with parsley and serve. This is a health- and energy-giving soup on a hot day and very refreshing for a baby who does not feel like eating. You can also add any of the following: debittered yeast, cooked brown rice, fresh courgettes, watercress, beetroot, apple, pineapple, grapes, almonds, or finely minced cooked chicken or fish.

SAVOURY MINCE

This is an excellent standby and, with vegetables added, makes a nourishing dish for either lunch or supper.

1 kg lean mince
1 onion, finely chopped
2-3 medium tomatoes, skinned and chopped
250 ml chopped celery
10 ml fresh thyme, marjoram, sage or basil, chopped
10 ml Brewer's yeast
2 carrots, grated
little oil
pinch of seasalt
10 ml honey
fresh parsley, chopped
water or whey from thick milk after you have made **CURD CHEESE** *(see p 57) OR 125 ml yoghurt, mixed with water*

Fry the onion in the oil until lightly browned. Add the mince and brown slightly. Add celery and tomatoes and stir in well. Then add the salt, herbs, carrots and honey and the whey or yoghurt into which the Brewer's yeast has been stirred. Add enough water to make it fairly soft and liquid and cook slowly until done, stirring occasionally and adding more water if necessary. Strain off some of the gravy to add to a small baby's vegetables as it is full of nourishment.

Serve with mashed potato, summer squash and mashed

green beans for a substantial midday meal. Alternatively, add a spoonful to scrambled eggs for supper, or mix with a little brown rice and stuff into lettuce leaf 'boats' or celery stick 'canoes'.

CHICKEN

Boil, stew or roast chicken and serve thin pieces that can be well mashed. Save the water if you boil it to make a nourishing gravy. This can be used as a consommé or chilled soup on hot summer evenings on its own. The water sets into a tasty jelly which can be used in vegetables, other soups or as a savoury jelly for a hot day.

FISH

Select unsmoked, unsalted, bland white fish. Always steam or poach it rather than fry it. Serve with vegetables and savoury white or custard sauce.

PULSES (dried beans, peas, lentils etc)

Soak all pulses overnight in water. Next morning, boil in enough water to cover. Toss in a sprig of thyme, marjoram or a piece of celery. Boil until tender in a covered pot, then drain, mash and add to soups, stews or vegetable dishes.

Mixed with mashed avocado and yoghurt, it makes a delicious dip or salad. This is an important food containing vitamins and minerals and can be added to any savoury dish. Serve with a little finely chopped fennel or caraway seeds to ease flatulence.

HUMMUS

This is a Middle Eastern favourite food and is delicious added to vegetables or spread on thin biscuits or bread.

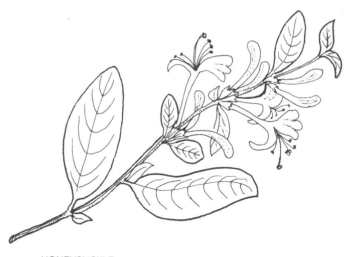

HONEYSUCKLE

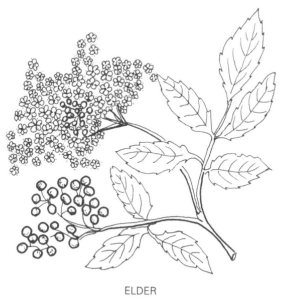

ELDER

71

250 ml chickpeas, soaked overnight
10 ml chopped thyme
juice of one lemon
25 ml chopped parsley
seasalt to taste
50 ml plain yoghurt
12,5 ml sunflower seed oil
10 ml fresh marjoram OR 10 ml chopped fresh mint

Cook the chickpeas with the thyme until tender. Drain and liquidise, adding yoghurt and other ingredients until a thick paste is achieved. Store in jars in the fridge.

GRAINS AND NUTS

Brown rice, barley, cornmeal and whole or crushed wheat are all excellent foods, some of which should be included daily in the diet. Grains can be boiled in water and the water used for soups and stocks.

BARLEY STIR-FRY

250 ml barley
1 ℓ water
sunflower oil
1 onion, chopped
1 tomato, skinned and chopped
2 courgettes, thinly sliced
10 ml fresh thyme, chopped
seasalt

Boil barley in the water for half to three-quarters of an hour or until tender. Strain. Save the barley water for drinks. In a pan heat a little oil, add onion and the barley grains. Add tomato and courgettes. Stir-fry, adding a touch of seasalt and the thyme (mint or fennel are also suitable). Stir well with a wooden spoon. Add a little water if it gets too dry and a tea-spoon of yeast extract. This makes a delicious light supper dish.

POTATO NESTS

6 medium potatoes
125 ml milk
25 ml plain yoghurt
12,5 ml chopped parsley

Boil potatoes in their jackets, then peel and mash. Mix in milk, yoghurt, a pinch of seasalt, and the parsley. Scoop into nests onto an ovenproof dish.

Filling

125 ml cream cheese
1 egg
25 ml wheatgerm
25-50 ml sprouts

Mix ingredients and scoop into the nests. Place under the grill for 5-10 minutes or until slightly firm. Serve with a slice of tomato, carrot sticks etc.

Cold fillings: Any of these will make a delicious light meal: grated cheese, tomatoes, cold cooked peas, finely chopped lettuce, celery, borage, comfrey, grated apple.

PULSE SAUSAGE

500 ml cooked dried beans, peas or lentils
1 egg, well beaten
12,5 ml wheatgerm
25-50 ml grated cheese

5 ml Marmite
few breadcrumbs
chopped parsley, thyme or mint

Mix all ingredients except breadcrumbs. Shape into sausages and roll in the crumbs. Fry gently in a little hot oil or place in an ovenproof dish, dot with butter, pour in a little oil and bake for 15-20 minutes at 180 °C. As a variation, add cooked minced meat or minced cooked chicken.

CHEESE AND RICE BAKE

250 ml brown rice, cooked
3 eggs, separated
250 ml milk
250 ml grated cheese, mild
25 ml wheatgerm
25 ml lemon balm leaves

Whisk eggs and milk. Stir cheese, wheatgerm and herbs into rice. Pour into a shallow baking dish. Bake at 180 °C for 20-30 minutes or until golden and set.

DIPS

Small children love to dip and lick. Try offering them dips of mashed avocado with a little lemon juice, or cottage cheese mixed with a little yoghurt and chopped herbs (eg borage flowers, nasturtium flowers, celery leaves, mint, parsley etc). Arrange a tray of some of the following to go with the dips: strips of carrot, celery sticks, sugar-snap peas, small tomatoes, slices of cucumber, pineapple fingers, apple slices etc.

CAKES, BISCUITS, BREADS

There is nothing quite like home-baked bread fresh from the

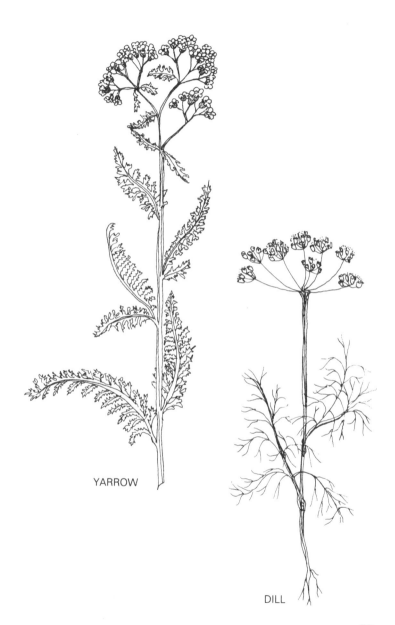

YARROW

DILL

75

oven. It is not difficult and can be a labour of love for your growing family. Remember though:

- Use only wholewheat flour or brown flour
- Substitute honey or molasses for sugar or icing sugar
- Avoid all sticky, sugary recipes. Seek out alternatives. (There are a number of tried and tested recipes in *Cooking with Winter Herbs* and *Summer Cooking with Herbs* in this series of little books.)

FRUIT BARS

250 ml stoned dates
250 ml dried apricots, soaked overnight in water
250 ml dried figs, soaked overnight in water
125 ml raisins
12,5 ml sesame seeds or coconut
180 ml almonds or pecan nuts
little honey to bind ingredients if necessary

Finely mince all ingredients, mix together and press into a greased tin. Leave to harden for about 6 hours. Cut into squares or bars.

FRUIT BREAD

12,5 ml butter
250 ml wholewheat flour
250 ml brown bread flour
15 ml baking powder
2 ml seasalt
375 ml milk
12,5 ml runny honey
25 ml molasses
160 ml seedless raisins

Grease and line two small loaf tins (or four to six miniature tins, or one large tin). Mix dry ingredients. Gently warm milk, treacle or molasses, honey and butter, add raisins and stand for five minutes. Add to the flour mixture. Mix well and pour into tins and bake for 20 minutes at 180°C (a little longer if using a larger tin). Serve buttered slices for a delicious teatime snack.

QUICK HEALTH BREAD

Get into the habit of baking your own bread. No bought bread can substitute for your own freshly baked loaf. This is my standard easy bread. I bake a loaf every day and it takes only 10 minutes to prepare.

500 g wholemeal flour
10 ml dried yeast
12,5 ml cooking oil
12,5 ml crushed wheat
12,5 ml sunflower seeds
12,5 ml sesame seeds
12,5 ml oats
7 ml seasalt
10 ml brown sugar
125 ml raisins
500 ml warm water

Mix the yeast with the sugar, oil and warm water. Add all the other ingredients except the crushed wheat. Grease a loaf tin. Spoon the mixture into the tin, sprinkle with crushed wheat, cover and set in a warm place. Allow the dough to rise level with the top of the tin (it takes about half an hour). Then bake in a hot oven (180 °C) for 40 minutes.

(If you like, sprinkle a little crushed wheat into the greased tin before you put the mixture in.)

SUNFLOWER SEED SWEETS

250 ml sunflower seeds, finely ground
125 ml ground almonds
125 ml finely minced prunes and dates
fresh orange juice

Combine sunflower seeds and almonds. Mix in prune and date mixture. Add enough orange juice to make a paste. Pinch off balls and flatten them. (Toss them in coconut if you like.) Place on a baking sheet and bake at 200 °C for two hours or until they are slightly crisp.

HALVA

250 ml sesame seeds
250 ml sunflower seeds
enough honey to make a stiff dough

Grind the seeds and add enough honey to bind. Spread into a container and keep in the fridge. Slice off squares or roll small balls in coconut. Keep in the fridge.

HEALTH ICE-CREAM

125 ml fresh cream
125 ml nut cream (see page 80)
60 ml honey
250 ml grape juice

Blend fresh cream and nut cream. Add rest of ingredients. Pour into ice cube tray and, when almost frozen, stick a toothpick or ice-cream stick into each cube. As a variation, try adding 125 ml mashed strawberries or peaches.

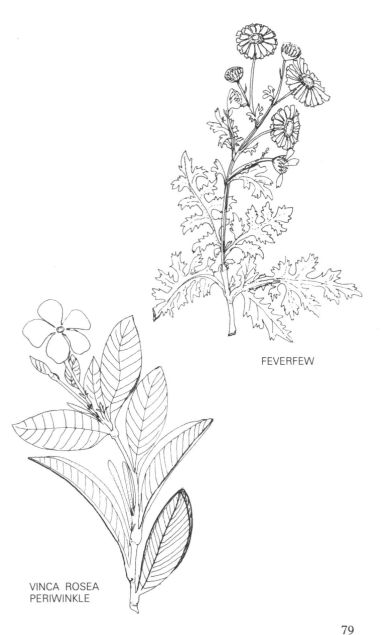

FEVERFEW

VINCA ROSEA
PERIWINKLE

79

NUT CREAM

125 ml almonds or pecan nuts, crushed
250 ml water
honey to taste

Blend nuts and water to a smooth paste. Add honey. Store in the fridge.

DRINKS

There are any number of variations in drinks for children. Fresh fruit juices are the healthiest and can be added to yoghurt, barley water, milkshakes and herb teas. I never put away my liquidiser while my children were small and, as they grew older, they learned to make their own milk- or fruit-shakes whenever they needed a drink. Try different blends, using melissa or mint herb teas as a base (standard brew). Add fruit, almonds, egg yolk, dried fruit, barley water or a little carob powder. Experiment and have fun – healthy fun.

FRESH FRUIT JUICE

Nothing can replace the nutritious and delicious benefit of fresh fruit juice. Invest in a juice extractor if possible and squeeze your own. Orange, pawpaw, pineapple and guava juice are only a few of the many fresh juices you can try.

CHOCOLATE FRUIT SHAKE

Blend a banana into 250 ml fresh milk. Add 5 ml carob powder and beat until foamy. Serve chilled.

VITALITY SHAKE

Whisk 12,5 ml nut cream (see above) and one egg yolk into

250 ml cold milk for a deliciously different milkshake. Add a little honey if you like and 10 ml wheatgerm to make it extra healthy.

ALMOND DRINK

Almonds and pecan nuts are suitable for children; avoid peanuts, Brazil nuts and pistachios until they are much older.

250 ml milk
12,5 ml ground almonds
12,5 ml ground sunflower seeds
10 ml honey OR 5 ml molasses

Whirl all ingredients in a liquidiser. Add half a ripe banana or half a ripe peach or 4 or 5 strawberries. It is the nicest milkshake ever!

HERB ICE-CUBES

When making ice cubes, place a couple of mint leaves, violets or borage flowers into the tray. Freeze. Serve with fresh fruit juices.

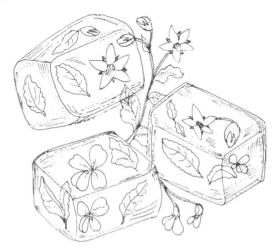

Treating common childhood ailments

Always work with your doctor when you have a sick child. The following are some simple tried and tested remedies for a variety of ailments commonly affecting children at one time or another.

Allergies
Stop all food that could possibly be causing the allergy. For two days feed the child barley water, bland vegetables (eg squash, pumpkin, potato, apple, oats). Herb teas (standard brew) will be safe too; lemon balm tea is probably the best to try.

Antibiotic
If your child has to go onto an antibiotic, be sure to add extra yoghurt (plain) to his diet, as well as B vitamins. Grapes, thyme and borage will all assist the body fight infection. Salads (liquidised with yoghurt for a baby) are important to help clean out the system; include a little lettuce, celery, parsley, fennel, cucumber and lightly cooked cabbage.

Asthma
Avoid all *white* foods (ie egg white, milk – for the time being – white sugar, white rice, white flour). Include comfrey in the diet and honeysuckle flowers steeped in honey. A pinch of

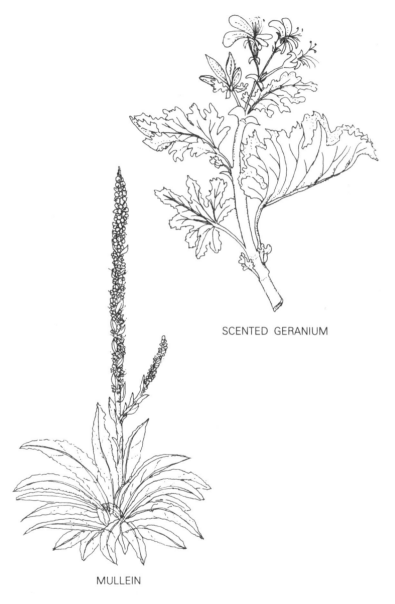

SCENTED GERANIUM

MULLEIN

83

ginger sipped in melissa tea is calming and soothing; mullein tea is also beneficial. Fresh fruit and vegetables are very important in the diet too. Oats are a good asthma treatment; give as a porridge in the morning and evening.

Bed-wetting
Pick one fresh thumb-length sprig of marjoram and one of catnip. Steep in 60 ml boiling water for 3-4 minutes. Sweeten with a touch of honey. Remove herb and give this drink to your child just before he or she goes to sleep. Start with 3-4 teaspoons until he gets used to it.

Boils
A warmed poultice made from a comfrey leaf, placed over the boil, will help to draw it to a head. Warmed pumpkin, oats, rue leaves or fenugreek seeds are also effective treatments.

Bruises
Make a soothing poultice using comfrey leaves, marjoram, fenugreek seeds or violet leaves.

Burns
Rub on the jelly of aloe leaves, or the inside of a banana skin. Comfrey ointment is soothing for burns too.

Calming
Melissa or chamomile tea are both soothing, as are teas (standard brew) made from celery, feverfew, marjoram or violets.

Carsickness
The day before you embark on a long car journey, make the diet light, ie no fats or heavy proteins. If you are setting off in the morning, serve a breakfast of oats porridge, with a little yoghurt and fruit, before departing. Avoid giving sweets or cooldrinks during the journey. Warm melissa tea with apple

juice is safe and soothing. Sucking on a wedge of lemon will help too. When the baby is old enough give him a mint leaf to chew. Ginger also soothes – add a pinch of bland herb tea. Try to keep a queasy child distracted and carry a facecloth, towel and water in case of accidents. If he should be sick despite all precautions, sprinkle the car upholstery with bicarbonate of soda to remove the smell.

Chestiness
Effective herb teas for a chesty child can be made using comfrey, mullein, sage, violets, maidenhair fern and melissa (standard brew).

Colds
Herb teas of comfrey, sage, melissa, thyme, chamomile, elderflowers, ginger, maidenhair fern and watercress will all bring relief. Hollyhock, violets and marjoram can also be made into effective teas. Olbas, a patent herbal medicine, available at chemists and health stores, is worth trying too, especially for a blocked up nose.

Colic
Herb teas of catnip, chamomile, thyme, caraway, coriander, dill, fennel, rue and sage will all soothe a colicky baby.

Constipation
Herb teas of violet flowers, chamomile and borage (fresh only), fennel, the mints, mullein, sage, strawberry, grapes (vine leaves and tendrils too) are all good.

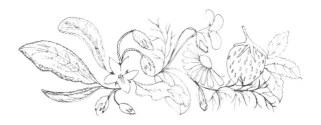

Convulsions
Your doctor should always be consulted. However, herb teas of catnip, chamomile and melissa are helpful. Also include celery in the diet, as well as comfrey, fenugreek, marjoram, mint and rue.

Coughs
Try a sage (fresh chopped leaves), honey and lemon juice mixture. Alternatively, thyme, honeysuckle flowers in honey, watercress, comfrey, elderberries, maidenhair fern, mullein, nettle and violet are all soothing.

Cradle cap
Make a standard brew tea using rosemary or southernwood, and use, lukewarm, as a rinse.

Cramp
Herb teas of chamomile, ginger, rosemary and lavender will ease painful cramps. Fennel, dill, the mints, parsley, pennyroyal and rue are also effective.

Cuts (minor)
Wash cut clean with a brew of rosemary, periwinkle (*Vinca major*), salad burnet or rosemary; then rub on aloe leaf jelly.

Diarrhoea
Flat Coke and cream crackers make an excellent remedy (the only time I will recommend a carbonated soft drink!). For a baby, whisk out the bubbles and mash the biscuits into the Coke to make them easier to take. A ginger herb tea is also effective. Include grated apple, raspberry leaves, mint and mullein in the diet.

Earache
Try Olbas, available from health shops and some pharmacies. It is a remarkable patent medicine for a number of ailments. Dab it behind the ear to soothe the pain. *Do not, however, put*

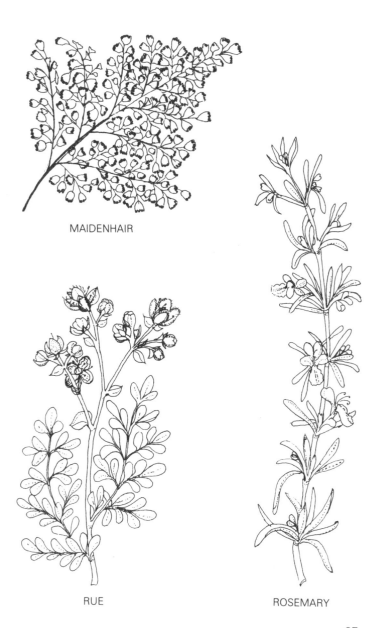

MAIDENHAIR

RUE

ROSEMARY

87

into the ear or nose. Mullein, marjoram and nettle leaves, crushed with hot water and made into a poultice, can be held in place behind the ear.

Eczema
As a wash or a rub use a tea made from either elder flowers, nettle, salad burnet, strawberry or oats (applied externally). Include plantain in the diet.

Fever
To bring down a persistent fever, try the following in the diet: borage, catnip, strawberries, the mints, raspberry leaf, cayenne, celery, fenugreek, hollyhock, lemon, rue, melissa, parsley, plantain, sage, and grapes (including vine leaves and tendrils). Frequent sips of herb teas or cool water will help too. Use the herbs in a bath of tepid water.

Fatigue
Raspberry leaf, comfrey, dandelion, fenugreek, ginger, pennyroyal and rosemary teas will put more energy into a listless, tired child.

Flatulence
Asparagus, catnip, caraway, the mints, thyme, dill, basil, coriander, fennel, marjoram and melissa are all safe and effective. Chew a piece, or make a tea.

Fretting
Soothing herbs for a fretful child are chamomile, melissa, thyme, dill, catnip, celery, lavender, oats and violets. Include in the diet and make into herb teas.

Grazes
Yarrow, plantain and rosemary will all soothe a grazed knee. Dab on or make into a standard brew tea and use as a wash.

Haemorrhoids

Comfrey, yarrow, feverfew, oats and plantain are good for this painful problem. Use as a poultice or as a brew for a wash.

Hayfever

Eat a little honeycomb every day, chewing the wax for a few minutes. Mullein and violets in a tea are also effective.

Headache

Rosemary, violets, feverfew, melissa, lavender, thyme, basil, catnip and ginger will soothe an aching head. Make standard brew teas and include in the diet.

Heartburn/indigestion

Fennel, caraway, the mints, melissa and sage will bring relief from the discomfort. Chew a leaf or make into a tea.

Hiccoughs

Try catnip tea or a teaspoon or two of peppermint tea. One teaspoon of honey in a little warm water also helps. A couple of drops of Rescue Remedy (available from health stores) will work wonders.

Infections

Asparagus, thyme, barley, carrot, ground ivy, lemon and sage will help fight infection. Step up intake in the diet. In the form of a tea, take ground ivy, thyme or sage as an alternative.

Inflammation

This can effectively be treated with any of the following: rosemary, thyme, comfrey, asparagus, barley, borage, comfrey, lemon or sage – take as a tea.

Influenza

Tea made from comfrey, mullein, barley, sage or violets will help fight flu.

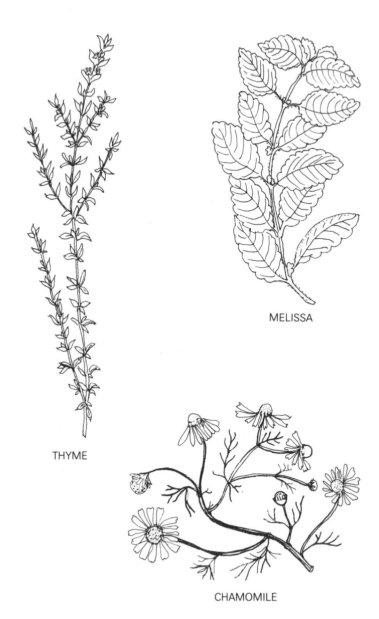

THYME

MELISSA

CHAMOMILE

90

Insect bites and stings
Rub on jelly of aloe leaves; a poultice made from borage, comfrey, mint or plantain will bring relief. For a *bee sting*, first remove the sting and then apply the inside of a banana skin to the painful area. For a *wasp sting*, dab vinegar onto the skin for instant relief.

Insect repellent
Place bowls of any of these herbs in the baby's room to keep insects at bay: the mints, pennyroyal, sweet basil, caraway, feverfew, southernwood, sage, lavender.

Jaundice
Include in the diet: asparagus, barley, carrot, dandelion and oats.

Kidney and bladder ailments
Violet, asparagus, celery, parsley, borage, ginger, lucerne, nettle, pineapple, southernwood, barley, carrot and comfrey will assist in clearing these conditions. Use as a tea, drinking at frequent intervals.

Nappy rash
A lotion made from either southernwood, elder, salad burnet or hollyhock are all gentle and safe for a baby. If the rash is bad, try to leave the baby's nappy off for a while each day. Lay him on a folded nappy on an old blanket while you keep an eye on him. Comfrey cream, applied daily, will keep him clear of rash.

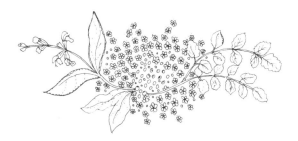

Nausea

The following herbs have a soothing effect on a queasy stomach: melissa, the mints, ginger, rose, basil, catnip, celery, coriander, dill, lavender, oats.

Nervousness

To calm a nervous or highly strung child, include the following either in the diet or as standard brew teas: melissa, rose, strawberry, catnip, thyme, celery, chamomile, comfrey, elder flowers, feverfew, lavender, oats, sage, violets.

Nosebleed

Yarrow or mullein: make a poultice of the leaves and hold against the nose until bleeding stops.

Pain

Any of these herbs will bring relief: catnip, coriander, feverfew, ginger, melissa, the mints, plantain, rue.

Rash

Children are prone to sudden, sometimes inexplicable rashes. Treatment with one of these herbs is soothing and effective: elder, southernwood, salad burnet, hollyhock, strawberry.

Sedative

Herbs which can calm a nervous or hysterical child, with no harmful effects are: melissa, borage, catnip, ginger, elder, marjoram, comfrey, oats. Make as a tea.

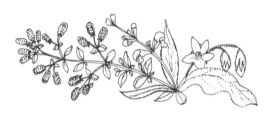

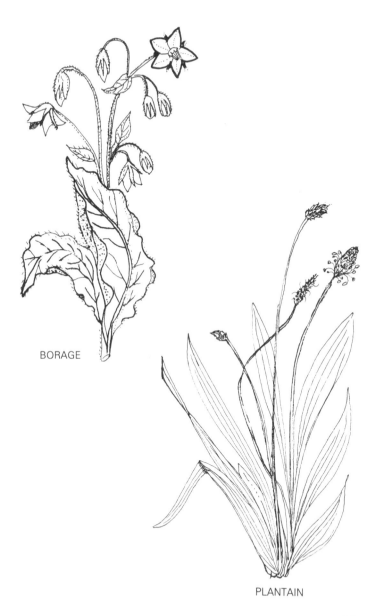

BORAGE

PLANTAIN

93

Sinus

The mints, pennyroyal, Olbas (available from health stores) or lavender will ease this uncomfortable affliction. Simply bruise the herb and inhale, or inhale the steam from pouring boiling water over the herb under a towel tent.

Skin disorders

Include the following in the diet: elder, marjoram, salad burnet, watercress, apples, lucerne, carrots, honeysuckle, lavender, plantain, rose.

Sleep

Sleep-inducing, soothing herbs are: chamomile, melissa, catnip, lavender and rose. Take in the form of a nightcap tea.

Sore throat

Sage and ginger will both soothe a bad throat. Chew a piece of leaf, or make tea of sage or ginger.

Sprains

Make a comfrey poultice with warmed leaves wrapped around the area and held in place.

Stomach disorders

Grated apple, and chamomile, the mints, melissa or mullein teas are all effective treatments.

Sunburn

Aloe leaf jelly, comfrey cream, salad burnet, waterlily stem (squeeze on the juice) will soothe effectively. Alternatively, dab milk directly onto the sore area.

Swelling

Make a compress from comfrey, borage, violet or plantain leaves. Warm in hot water first. Apply directly to the area, hold in place with a crepe bandage.

Tonic
In need of a boost after an illness, for example, include in
the diet: borage, rosemary, strawberry, catnip, chamomile,
watercress, sage, comfrey, salad burnet.

Teething
Dab Rescue Remedy (available from health stores) onto
gums, or two to three drops into the mouth. Include dandelion leaves in the diet for strong teeth. Oats, too, will help
build strong, healthy teeth.

Vomiting
Try Rescue Remedy (available from health stores). Basil, lavender, melissa or the mints can be made into soothing herb
teas. Sip frequently. Iced water with lemon juice is effective
too.

Warts
Dab wart frequently with fig leaf juice. The inside of a banana
skin, taped onto the wart and exchanged for a fresh piece
every day for 10 days, will be effective too.

Worms
Carrot, cayenne pepper, pumpkin pips and rue will all assist
in expelling worms. *NB Only use the pumpkin pip remedy from
three years old and upwards.* Chew 7 pumpkin pips first thing
in the morning (on an empty stomach) for ten days.

MEDICINE CHEST BASICS

Rearing children means having always to be on one's toes!
Nearly every day someone will need attention and you should
be prepared as best you can. Often treatment is necessary immediately until you can get to your doctor or at least talk to
him or her. Make sure, therefore, that your medicine chest is
always stocked with basic essentials. Always keep it out of

reach of your children. Have the following on hand:

- scissors
- tweezers
- cotton wool
- crêpe bandages
- gauze
- lint
- Elastoplast
- Bandaids

Rescue Remedy Dr Bach's famous drops can be used in an emergency and many a time they have been a lifesaver for me and my family. Health stores and some chemists stock them. I keep them in the kitchen, in the bathroom, beside my bed, in my car. They can be used for shock caused by any trauma, eg a fall, wound, fright, fear, burn, bite or broken limb. Just a few drops into the mouth and directly onto the affected area frequently gives you the time you need to cope with the emergency.

Olbas This is a patent herbal medicine for aches and pains, earache and blocked noses. Do not apply drops into the nose or ears; dab a little externally on the nostrils and behind the ears. It is good for insect bites, headaches and a stiff neck. Most pharmacies have it, as well as health stores.

Comfrey cream with Vitamin E You can make your own cream or buy it from a health store or pharmacy. My children called this the 'healing cream' as it rapidly heals all sorts of scratches, burns, grazes, sunburn and rashes.

Vitamin C For infections, for resistance to coughs and colds, Vitamin C is invaluable in the medicine chest. Take 250 mg daily, stepped up to 500 and even 1 000 mg in times of infection and illness.

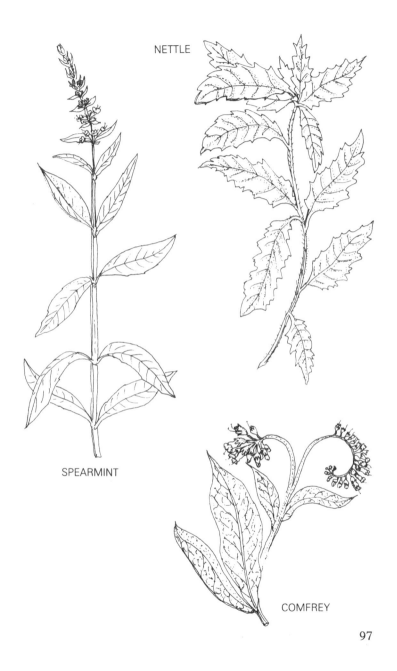

NETTLE

SPEARMINT

COMFREY

97

Now that you have read this little book, my hope is that my experience in bringing up my own three children can be of benefit to you. Experience, after all, is an excellent teacher, and I learned more about health in rearing them than I did in my hospital training.

May this little book start you and your baby on a road of glorious health and beauty. May it change your life and give you much pleasure as you watch your children grow.

For all that I have learned in the rearing of Pete, Gaily and Sandy, I must thank *them* for giving me such a rich, full and healthy life!

Bless all mothers – their task is a huge one, but one filled with much joy.

Margaret Roberts

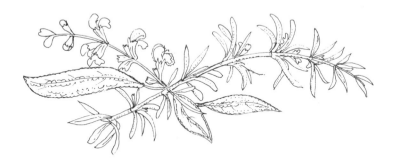

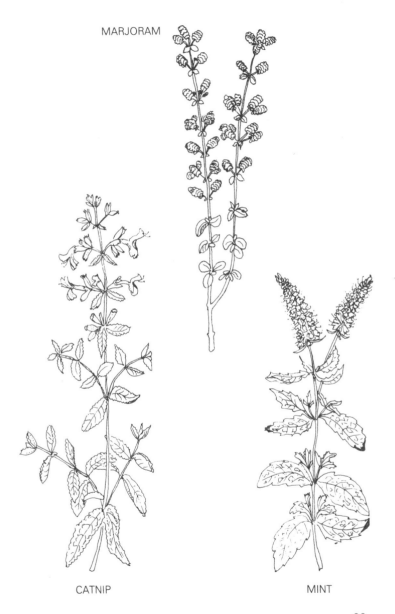

MARJORAM

CATNIP

MINT

Notes

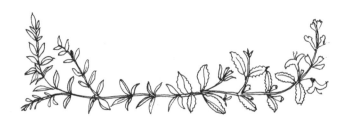

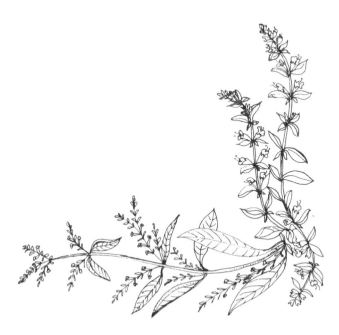

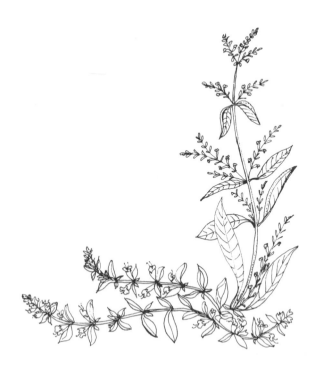

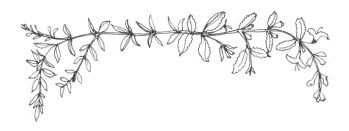

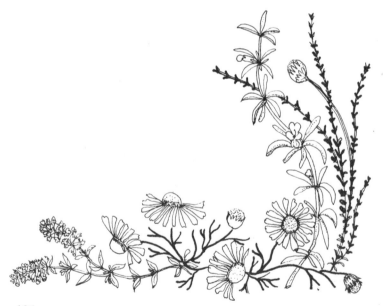

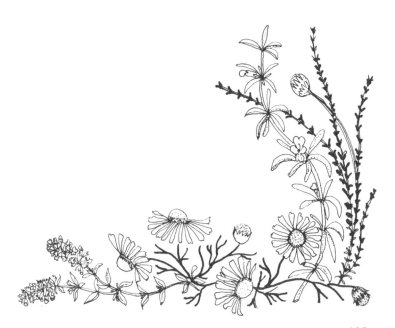

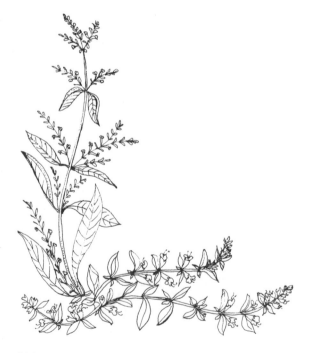

106